Introduction to Research for Midwives

Colin Rees
BSc, MSc, PGCE(FE)

Books for Midwives Press
An imprint of Hochland & Hochland Ltd

Published by Books for Midwives Press, 174a Ashley Road, Hale, Cheshire, WA15 9SF, England

© 1997, Colin Rees

First edition.

ISBN 1-898507-57-0

British Library Cataloguing in Publication Data
A catalogue record for this book is available from the British Library

Printed in Great Britain by Cromwell Press Ltd.

For Brenda,
and my sons, Michael and David

Contents

Acknowledgements

I have gained a great deal of enjoyment from teaching research to midwives for a number of years and was delighted to be invited by Henry Hochland to write this book. I would like to thank him and Catherine Bryant for being patient, and supportive while the book was being written.

I would like to thank Sandy Kirkman, School of Nursing Studies, University of Wales College of Medicine, who has had continued confidence in my ability to encourage midwives to be enthusiastic for research, both at degree level, and as part of the Masters in Reproduction and Health in Cardiff.

I have long been indebted to Chris Tucker for my involvement in Midwifery education in Bristol, and for Sheena Payne for my involvement in the BSc Midwifery course at the University of the West of England. All the groups in Bristol were particularly rewarding to teach, especially those in 1995 and 1996.

I would like to thank all the midwifery students in both Cardiff and Bristol who received some of the early drafts of chapters and 'consumer tested' them for me. I would particularly like to extend my thanks to Liz Hosegood, on the Masters in Reproduction and Health course, for taking the time to proof read a number of chapters very thoroughly.

I would also like to thank my work colleague and friend Ian Hulatt for his support and encouragement during this project.

Most importantly, emotional and practical support, as well as constant encouragement were supplied by Brenda Hauxwell, an inspirational midwife who has provided me with so much in life.

Finally, I would also like to thank my sons Michael and David Rees for their enthusiasm and support throughout the progress of the book.

Writing is an exciting but occasionally exhausting and demanding activity. The knowledge that so many people, including some I have not been able to name individually, were supporting me in this adventure was a great comfort and frequent source of inspiration. Thank you.

Introduction

Over the last twenty years midwifery has developed as a mature and potentially powerful force within maternity services. Many of the major professional and clinical developments have been underpinned by research. Yet for many practitioners research remains a shadowy, almost intimidating figure which is still surrounded by mystique.

The purpose of this book is to demystify research and make it accessible to midwives throughout the profession. The following chapters are designed to extend knowledge and develop a critical understanding of research in order to ensure evidence based practice. An attempt has been made to write in a straightforward, practical and purposeful way, so as to avoid reinforcing many people's worst fear that research is simply unintelligible jargon. Although the book should be relevant and useful to every midwife, it is particularly suitable for anyone undertaking a course which contains a research component.

The book integrates the following three themes:

- research methods and processes;

- the critical evaluation of research;

- the application of research to midwifery practice.

Each chapter outlines a particular topic, and raises key issues which need to be considered in applying it to practice. The relationship between the midwife and research is examined from two different perspectives; firstly the midwife as the 'doer' of research, that is carrying out research, and secondly the midwife as the 'user of research', that is critically assessing the research findings of others. These different relationships are clearly addressed at the end of each chapter under the heading **CONDUCTING RESEARCH**, which provides some practical advice on carrying out research, and secondly under the heading **CRITIQUING RESEARCH**, which outlines areas to consider in reading or listening to research reports. Each chapter ends with a list of key points which provide a summary of the main points.

Although textbooks are similar to other reference books and are not meant to be read like a novel in a sequential order, the book does start in Chapter 1 with a rationale for the importance of research in midwifery. Chapter 2 consists of some of the fundamental concepts of research which will provide the groundwork for the remaining chapters, while Chapter 3 outlines the basic structure of research. Once Chapter 4 on critiquing has been read, then the order of the other chapters becomes less important. However, reading is a personal activity, and you may find a different route through this book. If it is used as part of a course you may use it more like a reference book and just dip-in at strategic points. Whatever your reason for reading it, I hope you find it provides, if not the answers, at least an insight into what you are looking for.

One final word to emphasize is that this is an introduction to the wide topic of research. It is not meant to include chapters on everything you may want to know about the subject. A decision has been made, for instance, to exclude chapters on data analysis and statistical techniques, as there is only so much that can be included in an 'introduction'. Other topics and themes may also be felt to be missing. There are alternative sources available that cover these topics, and reference is made to these at appropriate points in the book. Those topics included, however, have been judged as essential components of an introduction to the subject. In particular, this book is built on the development of skills. This approach has been successfully used over many years of teaching midwives, nurses, and other health professionals, and it is hoped that you will find it successful here.

CHAPTER ONE

Why Research?

Does midwifery need research? Those who 'believe' in research will give a definite 'yes' to this question, while those who feel that on the whole they can manage without it will say 'no'. Research tends to be one of those subjects in which you either believe or you don't. Yet from a professional point of view there is no option; midwifery practice must be based on sound evidence and research is an important source of that evidence.

It is not easy to base practice on research. There is not the research available on which every clinical decision can be based. Even where research is available midwives may not be aware of it, or have easy access to it. There is also the issue of having a sufficient understanding of research to critically assess its quality and value. This is crucial if weak evidence is not to be mistaken for strong.

It is little wonder then, that in many situations other sources of knowledge rather than research influence action. In this chapter these alternative forms of knowledge will be examined and contrasted with the use of research based knowledge.

Sources of midwifery knowledge

What are the sources of knowledge you use to make clinical decisions? Think back to your most recent working day. As you think through it, list some of the things you did, and identify where you gained your knowledge on how to carry out that activity. The result should include some of the following elements which have been identified by several writers (Polit and Hungler, 1997; Lo-Biondo Wood and Haber, 1994; Burns and Grove, 1995; Talbot, 1995).

- Tradition (always done it that way)
- Authority/policy (told to do it that way)
- Education/training (taught/learnt to do it that way)
- Personal experience (found it usually works)
- Trial and error (tried several other ways first)
- Role modelling (seen others do it this way)
- Intuition (feels right this way)
- Research (the research I have read suggest this is the best method).

Some of these will be used more frequently as a source of decision making than others. It may be that research does not figure very prominently on your list. The aim of the exercise is not to make you feel guilty, but to sensitize you to the way in which decisions are influenced by sources of knowledge which will range in their accuracy and effectiveness. The list above consists of two kinds of knowledge; firstly, what Manley (1991) calls *'know-how' knowledge* (knowing what to do), and secondly *'know-that' knowledge* (knowing why you do that). Know-how knowledge comes from experience and practising skills. Traditional practice also often stems from 'know-how' knowledge. In contrast, know-that knowledge has a more theoretical basis and uses logic and an analysis of the evidence. It is research that is the only one in the list that is more closely related to 'know-that' knowledge.

Is research really better than the other sources of knowledge? According to Polit and Hungler (1997), research conducted within a disciplined format is the most sophisticated method of acquiring knowledge that humans have developed. The justification for this claim is provided by their description of the scientific method:

> 'The traditional scientific approach to inquiry refers to a general set of orderly, disciplined procedures used to acquire information. The traditional scientist uses deductive reasoning to generate hunches that are tested in the real world.'

This provides some clues as to the key qualities of research such as an *orderly approach* to data collection *in the real world* and the use of *deductive reasoning*. If we can clearly identify these qualities, they can be used as criteria against which we can compare the other forms of knowledge. Further definitions of the scientific method can be examined to develop this list. The following comes from the work of Feldman and Millor (1994) who outline the scientific approach as follows:

> 'The scientific approach is a system of logical and orderly elements that direct a formal, structured inquiry process in the effort to obtain knowledge. By combining several elements, such as logical reasoning, order and control, empiricism, and generalization, sophisticated systems of inquiry have been developed. Research is accepted as a scientific approach to knowledge generation when the processes that are used adhere to principles of logic, standards for data collection and analysis, absence of investigator bias, and rules governing generalizability or universality of findings.'

These comments on the nature of scientific knowledge can now be used to construct a list the characteristics that differentiate research knowledge from other forms of knowledge (see Box 1.1).

- An orderly and systematic process of gathering information
- Control over the process in which the information is gathered
- Objective evidence of a 'factual nature' taken from real situations (empirical evidence)
- Absence of individual bias
- Use of logic in analysing the information
- Can be applied to other settings (generalizability).

Box 1.1: Characterizations of research

These criteria can now be used to compare research with the alternative sources of knowledge used in midwifery.

Tradition

One of the big advantages of using tradition as a way of making decisions is that it requires the minimum of thought and its use is highly acceptable. As tradition suggests a procedure that has been carried out in a set way for some time, it seems likely that there was a good reason for choosing that option in the first place. It is also likely that traditional activities are acceptable to those receiving midwifery services, as they are likely to expect a certain procedure or solution to a problem. One definition of tradition by Behi and Nolan (1995) is that it is a practice that is constant over a long period.

It is not difficult to see the weakness of this source of knowledge; it does not necessarily mean that because a practice is accepted that it is necessarily beneficial. Behi and Nolan (1995) point out that procedures that are accepted simply because of regular and persistent use may have been based on an initial error, and subsequently accepted in an uncritical fashion. From the criteria list in Box 1.1, there is little to support traditional knowledge. Although it is sometimes applied to other settings and justified on the basis of its acceptance elsewhere, this does not provide sufficient justification for its use.

This basis for decision making has been the source of many research projects within midwifery. The routine use of enemas in delivery is a good example (Drayton and Rees, 1989). In this study the traditionally accepted practice of routinely giving enemas to women in labour in the belief that it would speed up the delivery was shown to be unfounded. Certainly many women have been very grateful for this type of research which has reduced unnecessary discomfort, and in the case of routine episiotomies, pain.

Authority/policy

The main advantage of basing decisions on policy or the rules and regulations of authority is protection against criticism. It is easy to justify decisions by saying 'I have no choice'. There is also the advantage for the practitioner in knowing where to find an acceptable answer to what should be done. From a service point of view, if people act in accordance with the current policy, then it is possible to achieve a common and consistent approach to activities. It is also a way of achieving control over what might be dubious or poor practices.

The disadvantage is that once policies are accepted they are rarely questioned, even when circumstances change. They become outdated and difficult to adapt because of the security people feel in following authority. Behi and Nolan (1995) point out that guidelines provided by those in authority may not always be as objective as we may think. Individuals may use their position to ensure that others conform to their personal beliefs or preferences. Accepting without question the word of those in authority, Behi and Nolan suggest, can inhibit the development of an open and questioning approach to professional activities. Feldman and Millor (1994) also agree, saying that both authority and policy guidelines must be considered and critically evaluated in the light of other sources of information, such as the literature and experts in the field.

Education/training

Education and training as the basis for decision making is very similar to authority, in that it provides a respected source of knowledge on which to base practice. We are professionally accountable to use only procedures for which we have been trained. It is easy to assume that if we were taught to do things a certain way, then there must have been a reason for it.

The disadvantage of this form of knowledge source is that it is difficult to move on and develop other ways of making decisions due to the strength of learnt and 'authorized' behaviour. Like policy and authority, education tends to maintain the status quo. People tend to do things the way they were taught, even though the information or technique could have been learnt a very long time ago. We have to remember that knowledge has a shelf-life, and there is a danger in following procedures and practices that have long passed their 'sell-by' date.

Personal experience

This source of information appears to support professional experience and individual initiative. We use this method of decision making in many situations, so it is a familiar strategy to us. However, personal experience does not necessarily guarantee that it is typical or correct. In other words, it lacks a systematic approach and may not be generalized to other situations.

Trial and error

This alternative seems quite promising as it does accord more with the criteria listed in Box 1.1. It can be described as an orderly and systematic process of collating information, and does collect objective evidence of a 'factual nature' gathered from real situations. There is also the use of logic in analysing the information. What is perhaps missing is the control over the process as the person carrying out such an activity may not try all the alternatives available and so miss a better alternative. Despite this, as Behi and Nolan (1995) point out, it can be highly regarded:

> 'Trial and error is a method that is used and often encouraged in nursing as a means of developing practical knowledge and skills. Unfortunately, the learner can assume something to be true on the basis of very few 'trials', often without confirming his/her belief with others. Furthermore, if widely accepted, such trial and error knowledge can soon constitute a new 'tradition'. Moreover, as a patient one would not appreciate, or accept being at the receiving end of such trials and mistakes, even if it may lead to new knowledge.'

This last point raises the question of ethics. Research attempts to safeguard the individual by including protection for those taking part in research, particularly clinical trials. Because of the 'ad hoc' nature of trial and error, the individual is not assured of similar protection. Feldman and Millor (1994) also criticize trial and error, which they refer to as a process of elimination, on the basis that it is inefficient in terms of both time and energy as it may take a long time to find a successful solution. In addition, they say, that solution may have already been determined by someone else.

Role modelling

Role models can be very influential in the way in which we solve particular problems. We might almost unconsciously adopt the solutions and approaches we have seen others apply. It has the advantage that it is an activity that is used by others and so has support. However, like so many of the other alternatives, just because someone uses a certain approach does not make it right. It could be outdated and not really applicable to the situation in which it is used.

Intuition

Intuition is not something that is characterized by an attempt to logically develop a solution on the basis of given information. It is something that occurs like a sudden flash of inspiration or insight. Looking at the list of the characteristics of research in Box 1.1, there is nothing relating to intuition that can be said to compare to research knowledge. It is almost impossible to justify or say on what it is based. This is illustrated by the definition of intuition used by Behi and Nolan (1995) who say it is 'acquiring knowledge without reasoning or inferring'. On this basis, although we may have some sympathy with intuition or sixth sense, it is not something we would expect to be the basis of professional activity.

The limitations of research

The conclusion we must reach is that research, as a basis for decision making, has so many more advantages than all the other alternatives examined. However, there are a number of points we must consider before condemning these other sources of knowledge. Firstly, we must remember that research findings may not be available to answer every midwifery question. Secondly, the research that is available may, for one reason or another, be flawed. Research findings should be challenged before practitioners change their practice. Thirdly, we have to remember that there may be situations where there is no time for the practitioner to consult the appropriate research. Rose and Parker (1994) remind us that applying knowledge to practice is not so cut and dried; it is often carried out in a very messy environment where the midwife has very little time to stop and think.

Where we do make decisions on the basis of these alternative sources of knowledge, we must acknowledge their limitations in comparison to research based evidence. If midwifery is to be taken seriously as a profession, to draw on the words of Walsh and Ford (1989), it must demonstrate that practice is not based purely upon beliefs, but rather that midwifery is a rational, fact-based discipline, more susceptible to change in the face of research findings and new ideas. The following final words are from Mason (1992), who sums up the argument for why use research based knowledge:

'In spite of the limitations, it is inarguably better to base our practice on research evidence rather than tradition: on science rather than ritual. The rigour of the research process generates evidence that forms a more accurate basis for the delivery of care than tradition, and consistency in care giving is more likely to be achieved thorough research than through habit.'

Conducting research

In designing a project, the researcher must remember the vital characteristics that make research so highly favoured as a basis for decision making. The project should follow the orderly and systematic procedures laid down in the research process (see Chapter 3). The researcher should take care to maintain as much of an objective and unbiased approach to data collection as possible. This equally applies to the way in which the results are interpreted. If these principles are followed, and if there is an attempt to collect information from a representative sample of individuals or objects, then the findings are more likely to be applicable to other situations.

In choosing the research topic, and producing a report of the findings, it is worth the researcher asking the question 'on what are decisions about this subject based at the moment?' It could be that if the answer is tradition, or personal experience, or even intuition, there could be a strong personal and emotional attachment to these current sources of information. This may produce resistance to change in this area, as well as a reluctance to accept the findings of research. There is not overwhelming support for research findings, particularly where they contradict firmly held views, or where their adoption would mean considerable changes in activity, and values. The relevance of this is that the researcher should anticipate the likely areas of resistance to the research from the start, and ensure that the design and implementation of the research take account of these areas.

Critiquing research

In examining published research, the reader should check the extent to which the researcher illustrates the characteristics found in Box 1.1. We need to ensure that the research has been conducted fairly, with as little bias as possible. We should feel that the information is objective, and the researcher has taken care in its collection and interpretation.

When critiquing research, some research findings may raise an emotional negative response within us, even to the extent that we do not believe the research, or we feel the researcher has 'fiddled' the results. What we are experiencing in these situations is a threat to our own value system, and the implicit belief in our own intuition or experience. We have already seen that these may not be accurate. In considering research reports, then, we should be aware of our own biases, and try to keep an open mind even where the findings contradict our own views and experiences.

KEY POINTS

- Midwives draw on a number of different sources of knowledge in order to make decisions. Some of these can be characterized as 'know-how' sources that are to do with knowing what to do, and others are to do with 'know-that' sources, which are to do with knowing why we do that.

- Although each of these sources of knowledge have their advantages, research has a number of distinct advantages over other sources of knowledge.

- Research is an orderly and systematic process of gathering information where there is control over the process in which the information is gathered. It produces objective evidence of a 'factual nature' taken from real situations (empirical evidence) where there is an absence of individual bias and a use of logic in analysing the information. Most importantly there is a greater ability to generalize the findings of research to other settings.

- As a profession demonstrating evidenced based practice, midwives have an obligation to seek out and apply the findings of appropriate research. We should be aware that research has its limitations but it is still better than basing practice on ritual and tradition.

CHAPTER TWO

Some Important Concepts

Learning about a new topic area such as research involves two processes; firstly learning and understanding some new words or concepts, and secondly discovering some of the issues related to those concepts. An issue may be defined as a situation where there is a difference of opinion over a topic, such as infant cord care, or a problem that needs a solution, such as how to increase the number of breastfeeding mothers.

This chapter will examine some of the important concepts used by researchers which often form a barrier to understanding research. An important starting point is to recognize that research takes many different forms. In this book we will distinguish midwifery research from that of other disciplines.

Midwifery research

So far we have managed to get through this book without defining research. There are a number of dangers in continuing in this way. Firstly, we will get to the end of the book and never discover what it was about. Secondly, readers may be forced to use their own definitions of the term, which means different people will have different things in mind. These various definitions may well not be the same as the author intended. We need, then, to give a clear definition of how it is being used in this book.

Research consists of extending knowledge and understanding through a carefully structured systematic process of collecting information which answers a specific question in a way that is as objective and accurate as possible. It has similarities to the process of audit, but goes further in the way it increases understanding and is placed within a context of professional knowledge. That is, it is usually placed within the context of other writers and researchers who have examined the same topic. Audit is usually interested in the performance of the service, or a part of it, and the comparison of results against an agreed standard or previous audit results which may allow action to be taken.

One of the simplest and frequently quoted definition of research is that by Macleod Clark and Hockey (1989), cited by Hockey (1996) herself as follows:

> 'Research is an attempt to increase the sum of what is known, usually referred to as "a body of knowledge", by the discovery of new facts or relationships through a process of systematic scientific enquiry, the research process.'

One problem in trying to define research is that it is like words such as 'care', 'delivery', or 'midwifery'; it is used as though it consisted of a single entity when if fact in can take many different forms. And this can lead to confusion. In the above definition, the word 'scientific' is used which may have connotations of people in white coats working in laboratories, when research can be carried out in many settings, and take a variety of forms and sizes. At this stage it is useful to think of research as a process which should conform to a number of principles, but these principles will change depending on the broad nature of the research.

In order to provide evidence based practice, the midwife may draw on research carried out by a number of different disciplines. Medical or obstetric research, for instance, will consider a number of clinical issues that will help the midwife both in terms of her own knowledge and action, and secondly in helping and empowering women understand situations that require action. In the same way, research from psychology or sociology may well provide illuminating information on how people behave and help the midwife in planning care. Research from education and the field of communication may also be relevant. However, the emphasis in this book is on *midwifery research*. This can be defined as research that tackles the problems and issues of direct concern to the midwife and which has implications for the work of the midwife more than any other discipline.

Quantitative and qualitative research

These concepts distinguish two very different approaches to research which are based on contrasting beliefs or philosophies regarding the nature of knowledge. Although each approach will be considered in more detail later in the book, it is important that we gain some understanding of the basic differences between them now, and their implication for midwifery research.

Historically, research has been synonymous with the word 'scientific', which is taken to mean objective and accurate. Its origins go back to the view that the natural or 'real' world is outside the experience of the individual and is open to study and quantification, that is, it can be measured in some way. This type of research can be characterized as *quantitative research* as it attempts to quantify elements, such as blood pressure, by means of a numeric value. These numbers can be summarized and may allow the use of a range of statistical techniques. This scientific view or 'paradigm' (model) of research is the one adopted by medical research as the right and proper approach for that profession. We must remember, however, that this is only one approach to research, and although it is useful in midwifery, there are other, just as legitimate ways of conducting a study besides 'counting' or measuring something.

Naturalistic research has a different view of the world from the above (De Poy and Gitlin, 1994). It believes the real world can only be understood through our personal experience of it. Everything depends on how we view it. This explains why some people are afraid of spiders or going to the dentist. It stems from how people experience them, or the associations they hold for the individual. It does not mean to say that spiders or dentists themselves are frightening. Naturalistic or *qualitative research* believes that if we are to understand a topic we need to look at it through the eyes of those who experience it, and try to understand it from their point of view. This type of research produces qualitative data and will use such methods as interviews or observation which attempt to capture views, opinions, experiences or behaviour.

Qualitative research attempts to encourage people to express their responses to questions in their own words. So, questionnaires with fixed choice options would not be classed as qualitative research even though they may have tried to see things from the individual's point of view. The reason for this is that the alternatives have been developed by the researcher, and the format does not allow the individual to express answers in their own words, only in those of the researcher.

An important distinction between quantitative and qualitative research is provided by the way in which the results of qualitative findings are presented. Although it is acceptable to present the themes found in the data in a table, showing how many people mentioned each theme (this is known as a frequency table), it is more usual for qualitative results to avoid numbers and simply present a broad theme heading and discuss the type of comments made, often with examples of quotes or dialogue. Both the qualitative and quantitative approaches to research are compared in Box 2.1.

ASPECT	QUANTITATIVE	QUALITATIVE
the research question	how much how many how often	what is the experience, feeling, opinion, pattern of behaviour
the type of question	precise requiring numeric answer	broad requiring verbal answer
use of hypothesis	for RCT's present at start	may emerge as a result of the study
issues/items described	through eyes of researcher	through eyes of respondent
data collection	extensive	intensive
sample size	large	small
sample	representative	relevant
extent results can be generalized	high	low
analytical approach	deductive	inductive

Box 2.1: Comparison between quantitative and qualitative approaches

Levels of questions in research

There is no shortage of questions that need to be answered through midwifery research. From the research point of view, it is the question posed by the researcher which acts as the aim of the research. In this book the phrase *'terms of reference'* will be used to mean the research question. The terms of reference usually begins with the word 'to' as in 'the purpose of the study was *to determine the effect of amniotomy on labour and neonatal outcome'* (Bannon, 1994). The section in italics would form the terms of reference. This is what the researcher 'refers to' when carrying out the study.

It is important to realize that research questions differ in their complexity and this will have implications for the structure of the study. Brink and Wood (1994) make a useful distinction between what they call the 'three levels' of research question. These levels are influenced by how much is known about a particular subject, or how much theory exists in relation to it.

Level one questions form the most simple level where very little is known about the topic. The purpose of this type of research is to describe a situation. The work of Bick and MacArthur (1995) is an example of this, where the purpose was to describe the extent, severity and effect of health problems after childbirth. The authors comment that little systematic work is available on the severity and frequency of symptoms following childbirth, and the effect they have on women's lives. Bick and MacArthur answer these questions in a level one survey and base their results on 1278 women who replied to a questionnaire.

Level two questions are those where some basic information is known about a topic, and there is an attempt to look for a possible relationship between two or more factors. Oakley's (1994) work on the role of midwifery support in pregnancy and its influence on birth outcome was an example of this type of question. In this study, midwives gave psychosocial support to a sample of women. The outcome, in terms of such measurements as birthweight, type of delivery and number of admission to hospital in pregnancy, was compared to a similar group who had not received support. This was an attempt to explore a possible relationship between social support and birth outcome.

Level three questions are used to test hypotheses based on already established theories about a topic. The work by Drayton and Rees (1989) would be an example of this. The results of their randomized control trial did not support the theory that enemas reduce the length of labour by reflexly stimulating uterine action.

These three levels form an important distinction, as they influence the type of approach the researcher must use to gather the data. Level one questions require a descriptive approach using perhaps survey methods. Level two questions require more sophistication in the method of analysis in order to suggest that relationships between variables may exist. Finally, level three questions require the use of an experimental approach which will test whether a hypothesis based on a theory can be supported by research evidence. Each level also requires more from the individual making use of the research as the amount of research knowledge and critical analysis increases in complexity with each level.

Variables

At this point we can examine some of the concepts that form the basic building blocks of research. Once we are familiar with their meaning we should find a difference in our ability to analyse research.

All studies are concerned with examining certain elements of interest to the researcher, such as pain in delivery, breastfeeding problems, professional updating and so on. The term *'variable'* is used to describe these items as they differ or vary in some way. For example, length of labour, attitude towards natural childbirth methods, social class, temperature, and level of pain in labour, can vary from one person to another. Burns and Grove (1995) state that 'variables are concepts of various levels of abstraction that are measured, manipulated, or controlled in a study'. We should, therefore, attempt to identify the particular variables of concern in the studies we examine.

In level two and three questions we can often subdivide variables into two types; *dependent variables* and *independent variables.* The variable that is the focus of concern to the researcher is the dependent variable, such as continuity of care, or level of pain. The variable that is presumed to play a part in influencing the dependent variable is known as the independent variable. An example will make this clear. Imagine that a researcher wishes to examine whether women who have attended antenatal classes feel more involved with their delivery than those who have not attended classes. The extent to which women feel involved with their delivery would be the dependent variable; attendance at antenatal classes would be the independent variable. The independent variable can be thought of as the influencing factor or 'cause' and the dependent factor is the outcome consequence, or 'effect'. Experimental research, which we shall explore later in Chapter 11, revolves around the examination of cause and effect relationships, where the researcher introduces the independent variable into the experimental group.

Initially, the difference between dependent and independent variables can be difficult to grasp. An easy way of sorting out which is which is to think of their chronological order, and identify which comes first and which comes last. The variable that comes first in time is the independent variable – the influence, and the variable that comes last is the dependent variable – the outcome. In the example above, attendance at antenatal classes happens before feelings of involvement in delivery, so attendance would be the independent variable, and the feeling of control, the dependent variable.

One danger in studies like this is that they appear to be based on the assumption that events are influenced by only one factor. Things are rarely as simple as this, and a number of other variables may influence whether a woman feels involved with their delivery. Other factors such as personality, the quality of the relationship with the birth partner, parity and social class may all play a part. These would also be independent variables which the researcher may need to consider. In any study, then, we should identify the dependent variable and the independent variable. We should then ask, 'is there anything else which could have influenced the outcome which has not been taken into account?' In this way we are becoming a more critical user of research.

Concept and operational definitions

These two concepts help us to understand exactly what the researcher means by the words used to describe the study variables, and how they were measured. The concept definition is a clear statement of the sense in which the researcher is using the words describing the concept. It is similar in some ways to a dictionary definition of the word. In our example of attendance at antenatal classes and feelings of involvement, although we may feel we do not need the words 'antenatal classes' defined, there are a variety of terms used to describe them in this country, and they may well not mean the same to readers from other countries. We would also be concerned about the concept definition of what qualifies as 'attendance at classes'. If someone attended just one or two sessions are they referred to as having attended in the same way as those who have attended six or eight? The other term we would want clearly defined would be 'feeling of involvement'. What exactly is meant by this? To provide an answer, criteria may be provided which specifies what counts as feelings of involvement. These might include whether options for intervention were discussed, whether the final decision was left to the individual, and whether questions and queries were fully answered and so on.

The meaning of the term operational definition is important from the data gathering point of view as it indicates how a particular concept is to be measured or 'operationalized'. Polit and Hungler (1997) define the operational definition as 'the specification of the operations that the researcher must perform to collect the required information'. So, for instance, condition of the baby following birth may be operationalized using the Apgar score which will permit different babies to be compared following delivery. Concepts such as pain are more difficult, but now pain scores may be used to operationalize level of pain. In a study of health problems following delivery, Bick and MacArthur (1995) asked women to mark on a 100 mm line how severe their symptoms had been for health problems they had experienced. This calibrated line is known as a visual analogue scale (VAS) and is used in a number of studies to operationalize concepts that do not usually have a numeric value attached to them. The line is divided into 25 mm sections so that the location of a cross indicated by a respondent along the line can be given a numeric value, and comparisons made between respondents.

Theoretical and conceptual frameworks

One of the aims of research is to add to the body of knowledge on a particular subject, and to increase understanding by developing a more accurate theory about why things happen the way they do.

A particular study cannot look at everything and will confine itself to a number of key factors or variables. The researcher's understanding of those variables can be expressed in terms of the theoretical framework which is being adopted for the study. This provides a clear context for the study. Burns and Grove (1995) define a theory as an integrated set of defined concepts and statements that present a view of a phenomenon and can be used to describe, explain, predict and/or control that phenomenon.

Bryar (1995), who is one of the few writers on midwifery theory, suggests that theory sensitizes midwives to the things that they should be watching for and helps to identify those factors which are central to care from those factors that are less important.

Theories can be categorized in several ways such as formal, informal or personal theories. An example of a formal theory would be Rotter's theory on internal and external locus of control (cited in Burns and Grove, 1995). This suggests that people differ in the extent to which they believe they can influence their own destinies and the things that happen to them. Those with an internal locus of control believe that they can influence to a large extent what happens to them. Those with an external locus believe that no matter how hard they try, it is those with greater power than themselves, organizations or even fate which dictate their destiny. The application of this theory to midwifery research would be to examine whether attendance at antenatal classes is influenced by an individual's locus of control. From this, a hypothesis could be constructed that those with an internal locus of control are more likely to attend because they will feel they can influence what happens to them throughout pregnancy and childbirth once they have the relevant knowledge.

Personal or informal theories are those beliefs we hold, frequently at a subconscious level, which influence our behaviour. We may encourage women to construct a birth plan because we believe that women are more likely to voice their own opinion if they have first thought about them, and then committed them to paper. The midwifery researcher may use a formal theory, or personal theory as the basis of a study.

Nursing research has been influenced to some extent by American nursing theorists, and studies have concentrated on such elements as adaptation, self-care, and stressors, as outlined in various nursing theories. However, it can be argued that as midwifery has different concerns and relationships with those with whom they are in contact, midwifery research should draw on midwifery concepts and theories. However, as Bryar (1995) points out, this is no easy matter, as midwifery does not seem to have developed its ideas as systematically as nursing. Although Briar does present five midwifery theorists on which it may be possible to develop midwifery research, four of these are American nurse-midwives, and only one, Jean Ball, is a British midwife. Interestingly, the key concepts of 'Changing Childbirth' (DoH, 1993), namely 'choice', 'control' and 'continuity', have been increasingly used in midwifery research as an organizing framework.

The relationship between concepts is sometimes presented diagrammatically to illustrate how the author visualizes the links between the dependent and independent variable(s). These diagrams are sometimes referred to as *conceptual frameworks* or *conceptual maps*, where key concepts are joined by lines and arrows to show the direction and nature of the relationships believed to exist. So a study may concentrate on the concept of breastfeeding, and be concerned with some of the independent variables which may influence the adoption of breastfeeding. A suitable conceptual framework which would illustrate the researcher's thinking may look something like this:

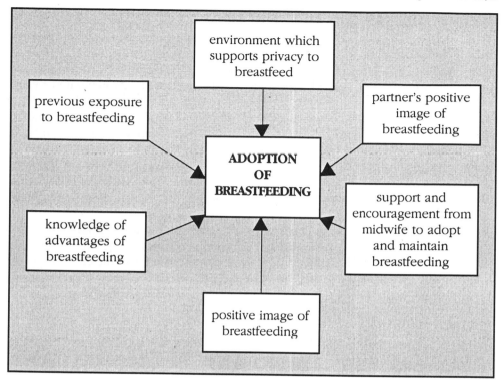

Fig. 2.1: Conceptual framework for a study exploring the decision to breastfeed

As can be seen, conceptual frameworks provide a mental image of what the researcher sees as the influencing factors or variables which will be explored in a study. This provides the researcher with a clear picture of the topic areas which should be included in the tool of data collection.

Polit and Hungler (1997) point out that not all research is linked to a conceptual framework, but where a study draws on one, then the design of the study, the key concepts, and the analyses and interpretation of data will flow from that conceptualization. In other words, they are a very powerful part of a research process. It is for this reason that a thorough review of the literature is essential to provide the theoretical and conceptual context for the study. This will then provide a clear indication of the key concepts to be selected, and possible concept and operational definitions.

One final word is that the use of theories and conceptual frameworks do vary between quantitative research, which will usually start with a theory and conceptual framework, and qualitative research which is more likely to develop one during or following data analysis. Remember, not all studies will make use of theoretical and conceptual frameworks, and they are not a feature of audit.

Reliability, validity, bias and rigour

These concepts may be familiar but their exact meaning may be unclear. Their use relates to quantitative research approaches and is concerned with the nature of measurement. *Reliability* relates to the method that is being used to collect the data and refers to the accuracy and consistency of the measurements generated by this method. If we wanted to measure the area of a room we wanted to carpet, using a meter length of elastic would make us distrust the reliability of the method of collecting the measurements. Reliability, then, is to do with the consistency of the measurement tool. If we were weighing a sample of babies, we would want to ensure any weighing scales used were first tested for accuracy. Where a number of different scales were used we would want to ensure that each one gave an accurate reading, otherwise the reliability of the results would be open to question.

Validity relates to what is being measured and is an attempt to ensure that the research tool is really measuring what the researcher believes it is measuring. So, for instance, we could think we were looking at the satisfaction of women with the clinical skills of their midwife, when we were really measuring the influence of the midwife's personality which may influence how women felt about the care they received. Although reliability is usually amenable to checking, and may become apparent in a pilot study, validity is far more difficult to confirm.

Bias

The degree of accuracy in the results of a study will be influenced by the amount of bias contained in the research. *Bias* has been defined by Polit and Hungler (1997) as any influence that produces a distortion in the results of a study. This can take a number of different forms, as we shall see in later sections. Here, we will concentrate on bias within the sample which may make them untypical or unrepresentative of the group they represent (see Chapter 12). This can happen through the method of selection.

In describing the sample the researcher frequently mentions the *inclusion and exclusion criteria* used to select those in the study. These terms relate to the characteristics of those felt to be typical of the study group – the inclusion criteria, and those characteristics that were felt may either put them at clinical risk, or which would introduce bias into the group – the exclusion criteria. It is important to examine these closely and assess whether you feel the researcher has attempted to control for bias in the way the sample was selected. Don't forget to also be beware if the study group or groups change for any reason, such as people dropping out of a study. This may make it difficult to carry on comparing groups, as they may no longer be similar in composition once a number of people have dropped out of the study.

Rigour

This concept relates to the overall planning and implementation of the research design. It addresses the issue of whether the researcher has carried out the study in a logical, systematic way and paid attention to factors that may influence the accuracy of the results. Burns and Grove (1995) suggest that rigour is the striving for excellence in

research and involves discipline, adherence to detail, and
that a rigorously conducted study has precise measuremen
sample, and a tightly controlled study design. They also
applies just as much to qualitative research as quantitative
methods, inadequate time spent gathering and analysing
quality of the research at risk. Polgar and Thomas (1995) a
the qualitative researcher is just as concerned with the soundn
they will employ different methods to ensure the accuracy an
results, as we shall see in a later section.

Midwifery is a discipline which needs to draw on both quantitative and qualitative research approaches. The issues and problems with which it is concerned relate to both the worlds of quantification found in the scientific approach, and the naturalistic world as experienced by those who come into contact with midwifery services, including midwives themselves. This book will concern itself with this wide spectrum of research approaches and illustrate how they have been applied to the concerns of midwives.

Conducting research

The key research concepts included in this chapter form the basic thought processes used by the researcher at the planning stage of a project. Understanding them is vital. It is like having a basic vocabulary in a foreign language that will allow you to cope with most of the situations you are likely to encounter.

The distinction between quantitative and qualitative research involves two contrasting broad approaches to research. In quantitative research, the researcher will design a study which collects information in numeric form, which may be summarized and manipulated using statistical techniques. Qualitative research, on the other hand, will mean the researcher will collect data, mainly in the form of words, either as the result of interviews, or observations. The approach used will depend very much on the nature of the research question, and what kind of data is implicitly implied in the terms of reference.

Similarly, the researcher must have a knowledge of the three levels of research in order to design the study at the right level. The level is based very much on the amount of knowledge already available on that topic. This means before the researcher can be specific about the level of the research question they must carry out a comprehensive review of the literature to establish the appropriate level of question required in the study.

The review of the literature should also help the researcher define the variables and provide a concept and operational definition for each one. Where the study is level two or three, the researcher should identify which is the dependent and which is the independent variable(s).

...g research

...articles can seem to be written in a foreign language, unless the reader has a ...nderstanding of the concepts introduced in this chapter. Once these have been ...stered the reader will not only understand far more, but will become more appreciative of good research, and will become more critical of weak research.

Knowing the distinction between quantitative and qualitative research will help anticipate the appropriate research approach, and the type of data collected. As will be seen in the next chapter, there are two different approaches to critiquing an article depending on whether it is quantitative or qualitative in design.

An ability to identify the level of the research question will allow the reader to make certain assumptions about the research and the form it will take. Knowing the levels also provides a way of critically examining the study to ensure that the researcher has conformed to the implications of the different levels, and has not carried out something which is inappropriate to that level.

In reading a research report, a reader should quickly establish the variables under scrutiny. The clarity of the concept and operational definitions will ensure the reader knows exactly what the researcher is looking at, and how it is being measured. Where the study is level two and particularly level three, the reader should identify which are the dependent and independent variables in order to follow what is going on.

The underlying theoretical or conceptual framework will also allow the reader to understand why the particular elements have been linked and the underlying assumptions that have been made by the researcher. In identifying the theoretical or conceptual framework, the reader should ensure that the items in the tool of data collection, and the discussion of the findings reflect the framework.

Critiquing is about assessing how well the researcher has done in designing and presenting their research. It is an assessment of both the strengths and weakness of a written or verbal research presentation. In order to provide a fair assessment, the reader must always keep the concepts of reliability, validity, bias and rigour in mind. These concepts provide an informed approach to assessing firstly the quality of the research, and secondly, the degree of excellence achieved by the researcher.

KEY POINTS

- Research depends on an understanding of some key concepts relating to how the researcher defines the topic(s) of interest.

- Quantitative and qualitative methods relate to the different approaches to research design, and are based on philosophical beliefs about the nature of empirical evidence. Quantitative research is based on the belief that information lies outside the personal views of the individual. It emphasizes accuracy, and produces numerical values. Qualitative research believes that knowledge is produced by our subjective experience, and that we need to look at things from our respondent's point of view. Midwifery is concerned with issues which draw on both approaches.

- Research questions can relate to three levels of exploration. Level one questions relate to describing one variable, usually about which little is known, or which has rarely been the subject of research. Level two questions look for relationships between variables but where little theory exists. Level three questions relate to questions where theory exists and the aim is to test hypotheses based on the theory.

- Variables are the elements in which the researcher is interested. In level two and three questions, there will usually be a dependent variable which is the outcome or effect, and one or more independent variables, which are presumed to influence or cause the dependent variable.

- Concept definitions relate to how the researcher defines the topic in which they are interested. This can be thought of as a dictionary definition or alternative word for the topic of interest.

- Operational definitions refer to the way in which a concept is measured. It reduces the vagueness of such words as comfort, and satisfaction by encouraging a clear specification of how they will be made visible for the purposes of the research.

- Theoretical and conceptual frameworks provide the context and meaning for the ideas and concepts contained in the study.

- Reliability, validity, bias and rigour relate to firstly the extent to which the tool of data collection is accurate and consistent between different measurements, or different researchers. Validity relates to whether the method does measure what the researcher intends it to measure. Bias is the extent to which the findings are distorted either by the choice of subjects or the method of measurement. Rigour is the extent to which the researcher has attempted to gain accurate results. This can be influenced by attention to detail throughout the study.

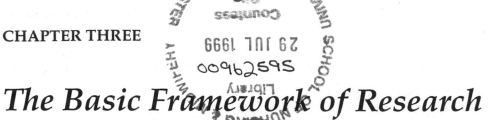

The Basic Framework of Research

An understanding of the basic framework of research projects is imperative, whether you are intending to carry out research or read research articles. This chapter will outline the stages involved in designing and carrying out a research project. The framework used here applies essentially to quantitative research projects; although qualitative research follows similar steps, the order of the stages may be different.

What is involved in carrying out research? There are two ways this can be examined, firstly by identifying the broad phases of a project, and secondly by looking at the more detailed stages contained within the phases. The broad phases of quantitative research have been outlined by Polit and Hungler (1997).

- **The conceptual phase**
  This is the main thinking phase where the researcher develops the idea for the research, and gradually develops a researchable question.

- **The design and planning phase**
  This includes decisions on the broad research approach and the tool of data collection.

- **The empirical phase**
  This involves collecting information and includes the pilot study, which tests the method.

- **The analytic phase**
  In this part the data is analysed and a report written.

- **The dissemination phase**
  Finally, the research report is communicated to those who can best benefit from it.

This outline demonstrates that research consists of a sandwich of THINKING – DOING – THINKING. The attributes of a researcher should therefore include an emphasis on analytical ability. This emphasis is supported by Sapsford and Abbott (1992) who suggest that:

'The key to good research does not lie in the techniques. Good research is the product of clear analysis of problems, clear specification of goals, careful design of fieldwork and thoughtful analysis and exposition afterwards. What lies between is just good, honest work.'

The essential feature of research is the systematic way in which it is undertaken. Like any process, it follows a sequence of stages designed to increase the consistency and accuracy of the outcome. Burns and Grove (1995) point out that a process consists of a purpose, a series of actions and a goal. We can now look at the broad phases outlined above in terms of the stages within them. The overall structure of the research process can be found in many texts and articles. Box 3.1 is based on a list of stages suggested by Rees (1995a).

---

1. Develop the research question.

2. Review the relevant literature.

3. Plan the method of investigation.

   This includes:

   a) the broad design i.e. experimental, descriptive, action, research, audit, etc.
   b) the sample, sample size, sampling method
   c) the information to be gathered
   d) the method of data collection
   e) the method of data analysis and presentation
   f) the ethical issues to be addressed before the study is commenced.

4. Carry out a pilot study.

5. Collect the data.

6. Analyse the results.

7. Develop conclusions and recommendations.

8. Communicate the findings.

Box 3.1: Stages in the research process

Stage one: The research question

Research begins when the researcher decides to carry out a study on a particular topic. Where do ideas for research come from? Perhaps one of the most common sources is the existence of a problem in the practice area. The researcher's first task is to take the problem and design the research question, or 'terms of reference'. This is a clear statement of the aim of the project. At the preliminary stage the researcher may think in terms of a question that begins with 'why', 'what', 'when' or 'how'. Brink and Wood (1994) call these words the stem of the question and what comes after them, the topic. An example would be 'why do women decide to give up breastfeeding?', 'What attracts certain women to attend antenatal classes?'. Giving up breastfeeding, and attraction to antenatal classes would be the topics and 'why' and 'what' would be the stem.

These questions are then converted into a terms of reference by removing the stem and replacing it with 'to identify', 'to compare', 'to determine' or similar phrase that outlines the aim of the study. So for instance, we could say the aim of our study was 'to identify the factors that influence women to give up breastfeeding', or 'to compare the characteristics of women who attend antenatal classes with those who do not'. Box 3.2 illustrates questions that have formed the basis of a terms of reference.

AUTHOR	QUESTION	TERMS OF REFERENCE
Hauck and Dimmock, 1994	what effect does a new breastfeeding leaflet have on the length of time women breastfeed?	to examine the effect that a breastfeeding information booklet had on breast-feeding behaviour
Floyd, 1995	how do community midwives feel about home deliveries?	to explore community midwives' experiences and feeling about undertaking home births
Paterson et al., 1994	what effect does low haemoglobin have on physical and mental health?	to assess the effect of low haemoglobin on the mental and physical health of postnatal women

Box 3.2: Examples of terms of reference

In studies at level 2 and level 3 (see Chapter 2), the researcher will usually state a hypothesis, or even more than one. A hypothesis can be defined as a testable prediction about the relationship between observed events (Polgar and Thomas, 1995). In experimental studies, the aim is to predict the nature of the relationship between the independent and dependent variables. A simple definition of a hypothesis is that it is the 'hunch' that the researcher has about the outcome of the study. Although hypotheses at level 1 are not required, as the purpose is not to test the relationship between variables, it is sometimes helpful for those conducting a level one study to consider what assumptions they are making about the factors that might influence the results, as this can help in the decision of what information to gather. So, in describing what attracts some women to antenatal classes and not others, the researcher might hypothesize that factors such as social class, age and parity may be influential. These would then be included as questions in the tool of data collection.

An important consideration at this stage is whether the question is researchable. Not all questions are amenable to investigation. Philosophical questions, or ethical issues, cannot be answered through research. Such questions as 'should midwives continue to wear uniform?' or 'should midwives reserve the right to strike?' belong in this category and are really the subject of debate not research.

Finally, it must be possible and practical to answer the research question. This relates to the feasibility of the research and concerns the availability of resources and expertise required to complete the study. Practical elements should always be considered when studies are being planned. Some of these have been highlighted by LoBiondo-Wood and Haber (1994) who make the following observation:

> 'The feasibility of a research problem needs to be pragmatically examined. Regardless of how significant or researchable a problem may be, pragmatic considerations such as time, the availability of subjects, facilities, equipment, and money, the experience of the researcher and any ethical considerations may cause the researcher to decide that the problem is inappropriate because it lacks feasibility.'

One of the most important criteria is 'will women and their babies benefit in a meaningful way?' It is crucial that we consider what should be included as priority areas for midwifery research. Allison and Tyler (1994) point out that in midwifery there is a need for research to be clinically relevant if it is to be translated into practice. They suggest a number of areas in midwifery where more research knowledge is needed. These include:

- The place and type of care given to women who experience problems during pregnancy
- Antenatal care that is geared to women's needs
- Evaluating pain relief
- Strategies to promote successful breastfeeding
- Prevention of incontinence
- Communication between midwives and women which allows women to determine the care that suits them.

The first stage of research, therefore, is a very complex. The type and nature of the question are all important, not only from the professional point of view, but also in relation to the research method. Many of the other stages in the research process will be influenced by the statement of the question.

Stage two: reviewing the literature

Studies should not be undertaken in isolation from previous research, therefore, the second stage of the research process consists of a critical review of the literature. The aim of this is to gain more information about the topic being examined, and clarify the research question (see Chapter 5). Although this stage comes second in quantitative research, in qualitative research the literature is not always consulted at this point, instead it is used at the analysis stage to help make sense of the data gathered. Qualitative researchers avoid examining the literature too early in case their own views are influenced by what they read, and so restrict the topics and issues included in data collection.

In quantitative research reviewing the literature is an important part of clarifying ones' ideas, and a necessary early stage in the research process. Midwifery is extremely fortunate in having such resources as the MIDIRS information system and the Cochrane data base to access information on published research. Local midwifery and nursing libraries, especially those with a CD ROM, are also part of the process of gathering information on previous studies.

The review is important not only to provide information on the topic, but also to provide guidance on the approach used by others who have studied a particular topic. The 'methods' section of research articles provide useful direction on possible information to be included in a study, and guidance on the way data can be gathered. Most authors provide some indication of problems 'encountered and comment on what they would have done differently with hindsight. All these are valuable to the researcher planning a study. Once this stage is reached, Bray and Rees (1995) suggest that the researcher stops, and asks the following three questions:

- Does it need to be done, or should we be basing practice on the research already available?

- What use will be made of the results? It is rarely worth putting a lot of energy into a project where there is little chance of it being implemented.

- Can I do it? Do I have the resources, skills and time for this to be carried out rigorously?

Unless the answer to these questions are positive, there may be very little point in carrying on to the next stage of planning the study.

Stage three: Planning the study

Once the first two stages are complete, the researcher is ready to plan the study from beginning to end. The quality of the research will be influenced by the amount of preparation and planning that has gone into it. Rigour is an important aspect in research, and is dependent on this thinking phase. Box 3.1 lists the considerations that should be included and consists of the following.

The broad research design

This is the blueprint the researcher will follow and is influenced by the purpose of the research. If the researcher aims to establish cause and effect relationships, as in a level 3 question, then the broad approach would be experimental. If the purpose is to describe a situation, as in a level 1 question, then a descriptive approach would be appropriate using perhaps a survey method. This may also be used where the researcher aims to identify if certain variables are related as in a level 2 question.

There are other approaches, such as action research, which is concerned with the introduction of change into the work environment and then evaluating its success and acceptability. This has not become a widely used method in midwifery, and there are few clear examples of its use, despite the view that its use is increasing in nursing (Holter and Schwartz-Barcott, 1993). The emphasis of action research on change makes it appealing to those who want to move practice forward. As it is a strategy designed to include those working in the areas affected by the change, it avoids change for the sake of change and ensures that there are benefits over the status quo (Webb, 1991). An example of its use would be the introduction and evaluation of a system of patient held notes.

Historic research is another method that has not really been used a great deal in midwifery, but is one that may provide a sense of development within the profession. It relies on the use of historical records and accounts, such as diaries, to chart the course of a particular issue or problem. The work of Kirkham (1995) is one example where documents, reports and Government papers relating to midwifery supervision have been examined to analyse the way supervision has developed.

Finally, audit has been included as a broad research approach. Although not strictly research, the use of audit in midwifery has become so common that it merits inclusion. Audit requires the same systematic approach and rigour found in research. It does not necessarily have the intention of adding to midwifery knowledge, nor can the results of one audit be applied elsewhere, yet it does answer important questions that are very similar to level 1 research questions.

The sample

The sample relates to the people, items, or events included in the research (see Chapter 12). In the planning stage the researcher must consider the characteristics that make individuals eligible for selection, and those which would make them unsuitable or even put them at risk or at a disadvantage. These form the inclusion and exclusion criteria of the study. The researcher should also attempt to estimate the intended size of the sample. Comparisons with previous research may provide some clues as to optimum size, as well as helping with the sampling method.

The specific information to be collected.

In any study it is tempting to collect information simply for the sake of it, out of a belief that everything is relevant and should be included. This will result in information overload and make it difficult to do anything with the findings. The researcher should consider each item to be included and ask two questions:

* Is this relevant to my terms of reference?
* What use am I going to make of this information?

Unless both of these can be clearly answered the information should not be included.

The method of data collection

There are a number of alternative tools of data collection that can be used to gather information. The most frequently used ones can be listed as:

- Questionnaires
- Interviews
- Observation
- Documentary methods
- Experimental methods.

Each one will have its advantages and disadvantages, so how does a researcher know which one to choose? One of the main considerations in selecting the data collection tool is the terms of reference. If the research question is related to staff or women's experiences, views and opinions, and they are in the best position to provide an answer, then questionnaires or interviews will be appropriate. Where the researcher is interested in behaviour or technique, such as the technique of suturing, then observation will be a more reliable method. This is true of any question where we are concerned with what people do, rather than with what people say they do. Remember too, that much of our behaviour and actions are so automatic and carried out at a subconscious level, that we may find it difficult to accurately describe what we do. For standard quantitative data, midwifery notes or the medical record may be the best source of information. Finally, where we are carrying out a level 3 study where we want to examine the existence of cause and effect relationships, we would use experimental methods.

It is possible to use more than one method in a single study and this is called *triangulation.* It is used to overcome the limitations of a single method of collecting data and so increase the validity of the results. As part of triangulation, researchers might interview midwives on how they discuss smoking in pregnancy with mothers, and then observe interactions to provide a fuller picture of what goes on.

The method of analysis and presentation

Whichever method is selected to gather the data, the method of analysis should be considered at the design stage. If the analysis will involve the use of statistics, then the researcher must decide which statistical techniques would be most appropriate, or consult someone who can provide advice. At this stage it is also important to think how the results will be presented, especially if one item of information is to be cross-tabulated with another. An example would be where the method of infant feeding is to displayed by parity. The method of analysis will also influence the form in which the information is collected. If the researcher wanted to provide an analysis of the average length of time babies were breastfed, it would be necessary to ask women for the time in weeks and not ask them to tick a box that related to a spread of weeks, for example 3–6 or 7–10 weeks, as averages are calculated on individual figures and not a range.

Ethical issues

Just as the midwife is bound by a professional code of conduct, so the ↘
bound by an ethical code in conducting research. Ethics in research relate to a ↘
of issues that include the following:

- Informed consent
- Confidentiality
- The avoidance of harm or exposure to risk
- The avoidance of raising expectations which it may not be possible to meet
- The use of a local research ethics committee (LREC) where appropriate to approve the study.

All of these issues are covered in Chapter 7. At the planning stage the researcher must consider the implications of the study for each of these issues and ensure they have been addressed.

Once the planning is complete the researcher may produce a *research protocol*. The term proposal is also used to describe the same thing (Wraight, 1995). This is a written outline of the study and includes the justification for the study, the terms of reference and many of the details developed in the planning phase. The research protocol may be used to gain permission to undertake the study, gain funding or submitted to the ethics committee, if appropriate, to gain ethical approval. The production of a protocol is also invaluable to the researcher as it allows them to assess their ideas on paper. This may reveal some problematic aspects of the study that had not been apparent previously.

Stage four: Pilot

Before the study is carried out, the researcher must ensure that there are no unanticipated problems in gaining access to the data, and that the method used to collect the data will work. This is the role of the pilot study. Polit and Hungler (1997) define the pilot as a small-scale version, or trial run, of the major study. Although its purpose is usually thought to relate to checking the accuracy of the data collection tool, it should be used to consider a range of factors. The whole feasibility in terms of the resources, time, the availability of subjects for the study, their willingness to participate and the support required from others to facilitate data collection, all need to be assessed before a total and perhaps expensive commitment to the study is made.

The results gathered in the pilot should also be analysed to test the way they will be processed in the main study. The major purpose will be to assess the reliability of the tool and to provide the researcher with experience and practice in using it. Refinements can then be made which will allow the main study to progress as efficiently as possible. In this way the pilot study is very much like a dress-rehearsal that allows all the elements in the study to be tested and adjustments made before the opening night.

Stage five: Data collection

Once the pilot had been completed the researcher is in a position to start data collection. As can be seen, this comes quite some way into the total process. Bray and Rees (1995) warn that although the researcher tries to anticipate problems, unexpected things do go wrong. Postal strikes happen once questionnaires have been sent out and delay their return; sickness and absence reduce the number of staff available for interview; newspapers and television suddenly promote the very topic being measured as part of the knowledge of those in contact with services. All this is inevitable and a normal part of the research process.

Stage six: Data analysis

Data analysis takes place when the data has been collected. This consists of counting, classifying, and grouping the individual pieces of data so that a broad pattern may be discernible. Descriptive statistics may be used to present a picture of the results using techniques such as averages (Clegg, 1982). Tables and graphs are used to show the results in a visually informative way. Statistical tests or correlation may be used to establish if there are any statistical associations present (Clegg, 1982). In qualitative research the vast amount of information collected is analysed to establish themes. This is the process of content analysis (Morse and Field, 1996). These themes are then compared with the literature to achieve greater validity of the findings, and to help in theory construction.

Stage seven: Conclusions and recommendations

The data analysis should lead to conclusions. These should be based on and supported by the results. The conclusion should also provide an answer to the terms of reference, and, where appropriate, say whether the study hypothesis has been accepted or rejected (we do not say proved or disproved because it is usually difficult to be that certain. There is always the possibility of a margin of error). The implications of the findings are then discussed and will result in some recommendations both for further research and for changes in practice where appropriate.

Stage eight: Communication of findings

Research will only be useful if it is communicated. The last stage in the research process consists of the production of a report, article or verbal presentation where the author will provide the following details:

- What they set out to do
- Why they did it
- How they did it
- What they found
- What it all means.

We can now use this knowledge of the research process in the next chapter which covers how to critiquing research articles and reports. Further chapters will look at some of the topics and issues covered in this chapter in more detail.

Conducting research

This chapter has presented the basic framework the researcher must follow in carrying out research. This is very systematic and has an internal consistency where every stage has implications for further stages. Although it is presented here as a series of steps, it should be acknowledged that some of these are carried out in parallel or the researcher may go back to certain stages. It is not necessarily as neat as it appears.

The essence of good research is planning, and the researcher will considerably increase their chances of a successful project the more time they spend on this stage. The importance of the review of the literature as a source of information and ideas on the research approach should also be emphasized. Above all, the researcher should not be tempted to cut corners by neglecting a pilot study, as so many unanticipated problems can be revealed at this stage.

The feasibility of the study should be carefully considered, and two important elements at the planning stage are firstly to think about permission to conduct the study, and secondly to design the method of data analysis, particularly where this may involve statistics. Where the study may need ethical approval it is worth contacting the appropriate Local Research Ethics Committee (LREC) as soon as possible, as this can seriously delay a study where such committees meet irregularly, or where they have to deal with large numbers of applications. A research protocol, which is the outline of the intended research, will have to be submitted (Wraight, 1995), and it is worth getting advice from someone who may have experience in this. Similarly, at this stage advice should be sought from someone who had an understanding of statistics, and the analysis of data. This will have a profound effect on the type and format of the information included in the data collection tool. A mistake at this point could mean that a large part of the information collected is unusable because it has not been collected in the right way.

Although researchers can spend a great deal of time on planning, and even on piloting the study, it should always be remembered that inevitably things do not always run smoothly, and the unexpected may well happen to you. Research is a skill acquired over time through experience. Don't give up when things go wrong, adjust your plan.

Critiquing research

The research process framework provided in this chapter gives a clear structure against which projects can be evaluated. As you read through a research report there should be clear evidence that the stages in the research process have been followed, and the issues outlined in this section addressed. If they have not, then you are justified to cast doubt on the way the researcher has conducted the study. Remember, however, that qualitative research has a different structure, and will look different in comparison to quantitative research reports.

When critiquing a study, the important question is has the researcher followed a sensible structure for the study, given the nature of the research question? Following this, the next question should be, does each decision fit with the previous decision made in the process? Once you are familiar with the stages of research you will begin to see the structure clearly evident in the reports you read. The next chapter will help you develop a more challenging approach to your critique.

KEY POINTS

- Research projects are structured around a number of stages that give the researcher a path to follow. The aim of this framework is to increase objectivity, reliability, validity and the rigour of the research.

- The exact sequence of steps will vary depending on the broad research design, so qualitative research is different from quantitative.

- Knowing these steps enable the reader of a research project to assess whether the correct stages have been followed.

CHAPTER FOUR

Critiquing Research Articles

The main purpose of midwifery research is to increase the quality of care through the application of knowledge gained from systematic data collection and analysis. There is a problem, however, and that is the quality of research does vary. We must remember that there is rarely such a thing as the perfect research project. Researchers seldom have ideal conditions in which to carry out their work. One definition of research is that it is making the best of a bad job. But how does the midwife who reads research know what is a good research, and which should be treated with caution?

Critiquing research is part of the answer. A critique is a careful consideration of both the strengths and limitations of published research. It is on the basis of this that the reader can consider the implications for practice. Although the word critique is often linked with the word criticize, Talbot (1995) points out that a critique is meant to be constructive and not punitive. In other words, a balanced view is imperative. It is a way of using critical skills to reflect on, not only the whole process in which the research was undertaken, but also the thinking that lies behind the research.

Critiquing is a skill that requires practice. First of all, it requires a knowledge of how to critique. As Polit and Hungler (1997) observe, it is not just a review or summary of a study, but rather a careful, critical appraisal of the strengths and limitations of a piece of research. The aim of this chapter is to provide a structure for critiquing research articles.

As quantitative research is different to qualitative research, the first framework will relate mainly to quantitative research. A second framework for qualitative research will be presented later in the chapter. Some of the details within both structures are based on information in later chapters. This means that you may need to look at later chapters for more detail on some of the points. The skill of critiquing is presented at this point in the book as it should be started early in the process of developing an understanding of research.

As you read this chapter, have a research report that is not too complex by your side. This will help you become familiar with applying the structure of a critique. In the first section you will need an example of quantitative research, where the results are presented in the form of numbers, and in the second part a piece of quantitative research where broad themes, and dialogue or quotes are used. There are many examples of qualitative research available, but a good and accessible example of quantitative research would be Bluff and Holloway (1994), or Davies (1996). An excellent longer piece of qualitative research is Hunt and Symonds (1995).

Applying the critiquing framework

When faced with a research article, the reader should consider the following three questions:

1. What does it say?
2. Can I trust it?
3. How does it contribute to practice?

The first question relates to *comprehension*, and is concerned with such elements as what did they look at? Why did they look at it? How did they go about it? What did they find? What conclusions did they come to? The second question relates to an *assessment* of the research process in terms of rigour – how well was it thought through, and what steps were taken to reduce problems of bias, reliability and validity? This second question requires a knowledge of some of the issues and techniques of research which will be covered throughout this book. The third question relates to an *evaluation* of the study's contribution to professional practice – does it provide clear evidence for changing or challenging practice? Who might benefit, and in what way, from the study?

If we start with the first question of comprehension and what it says, we might feel that if we read it through we will know what it says. This is not necessarily the case. We know from experience that our reading style may cause us to be selective in what we remember from written material. We will tend to recall unusual or interesting details, or pick out information that reinforces our own views on issues. In other words, our uncritical and unstructured approach to reading may mislead us in our recollections and assessments of written material.

Our very reading style can also make it difficult to accurately assess an article. For instance, have you ever started to read a page of an article, and started at the top of a column, but by the time you have reached the bottom you have no recollection of what you read at the top? If that is a familiar feeling you are in good company. Most of us read passively a great deal of the time. Reading research articles is very different from reading a novel. In fiction the writer is continually drawing pictures in our minds and influencing our feelings, as well as perhaps our senses, with descriptions of sounds, smells and emotions. Research writing is not like that. It requires an approach that is far more active and analytical.

To help us improve our active reading skills and our analytical faculties, we need two things; first of all we need to divide the article into its component parts. This will allow us to see the overall outline of the research, and understand how all the pieces fit together. Secondly, in order to be an active reader it will help us if we have a list of questions to which we can actively search out answers. Box 4.1 provides such a framework and list of questions. The following sections will now look at these headings in detail.

Focus and background

When reading a research article the first thing we need to do is identify the broad area it covers, so we can put it in the context of existing knowledge. The *focus* of an article provides a clue to the general topic it covers. This should be expressed in a few words that include the key concepts covered in the article. These might be found in the title, and most certainly in the terms of reference. Ask yourself what is the basic theme of this article? The answer might be 'empowering women to make informed choice', 'care of the perineum', or 'effectiveness of postnatal visits'. Notice that these are not questions, nor are they long and detailed. We are looking at the broad canvas of which this study forms a part. It should be stressed that with the focus there is not a clear right or wrong answer, it depends very much on what you see as the basic purpose of the article. Some articles might be put under the focus of 'communication problems', or 'assessing change', while others may be more narrow, such as 'the reduction of pain in labour'.

The *background* to a study answers the question 'how does the researcher justify choosing this topic area?' Here we should expect to see a clear argument as to why the topic is a problem, the nature and implications of that problem, and how it has been approached in the literature. A study should start with the identification of a problem.

The author may use the subheading *'review of the literature'* in which previous work will be examined. Some articles will contain only a summary or synopsis of previous work. Where possible, however, an author should provide a critical review of the literature. This should draw attention to both strengths and weakness, of individual works, and the literature overall. In this section the author may explicitly or implicitly draw together the theoretical or conceptual framework of the study. Which concepts or variables are seen as linked for the purpose of this study?

All of this should prepare the way for the *terms of reference* which will say how the problem is to be explored in this particular study. There are two places where the terms of reference can usually be found. The first is in the summary sometimes found underneath the title, or in the margin in some journals. The second place is just before the subheading 'method'. Although the terms of reference usually begin with the word 'to', sometimes we need to insert it ourself because of the grammatical construction of the sentence. If the work is experimental there might also be a *hypothesis*. Both the terms of reference and hypothesis will be important as our evaluation of some elements of the method, and particularly the conclusion, will be influenced by the author's stated intention of what they wanted to find out, or test.

With the terms of reference and the hypothesis, if present, it should be possible to identify which of the three levels of research questions has been used (see Chapter 2). The variable or variables should also be evident at this stage. Where the question is level 2 or 3, what are the dependent and independent variables? Has the author provided satisfactory concept and operational definitions for the variables?

Throughout all these sections it is important to keep to the author's own words rather than paraphrase them, as we could change their meaning. In critiquing, it is also important that we are doing two things; we should not only be describing the content under one of the headings in the critique framework, but we should also say how well the author has accomplished that element. In other words it is not simply what they said, but how well did they say it?

Methodology

In this section of the critique the reader's task is to identify the structure of the project, and whether the *design* is a suitable choice to answer the question. The first stage is to identify the broad research approach in terms of is it an experimental design with an experimental and control group, is it correlation where the researcher is searching for factors which appear together, not necessarily in a cause and effect relationship, is it a survey where the purpose is description, or is it action research which involves the introduction of change but with no control group? The important point here is whether a suitable design has been chosen.

Within the broad research approach, which *tool of data collection* has been used? We should consider some of the strengths and weakness of the method chosen in order to judge whether the author has chosen wisely. Is there recognition of some of the limitations of that method? Has triangulation been applied where the author has used more than one tool of data collection? We would also consider whether the researcher has attempted to reduce the problem of reliability. For instance, have they used a pilot study to check the consistency of the tool of data collection?

The critique includes not only an assessment of the tool of data collection, but the *ethical issues* related to its use. Here, we are looking for a recognition that informed consent, confidentiality, and an evaluation of the possible negative consequences of taking part in the study, are an important part of the research process. Has the study been approved by an ethics committee, or is it not appropriate in this case? (see Chapter 7)

We should also look closely at the *sample* of people, events or objects involved in the study. Are there clear inclusion and exclusion criteria that will help us consider were they appropriate for the study (see Chapter 12)? We should also identify the total numbers on whom the results are based. Here, we need to be careful, as large numbers could be initially involved but through poor response, individuals dropping out, or being eliminated from analysis for one reason or another, the final numbers could be quite small. Our main concern with the sample is whether we feel that it is representative of the group they represent. It is not only sample size, but geographical variations, and characteristics of the sample that we need to think about. Where people are involved, could there be cultural patterns related to the part of the country or social class that might also influence the results?

Findings

In this section we are concerned with the data the researcher collected, the way it is presented and the extent to which it answers the terms of reference. It is important to make the distinction between the main findings of a study, and what we might think of as interesting findings. We need to limit our view of the main findings to those results that might have a reasonably large number attached to them, and which relate to the terms of reference. We do have to consider what might be an appropriate or anticipated response to questions or measurements, against which we can compare the actual findings. For example, what proportion of women would we expect to have the same midwife present throughout labour? If we would expect in the region of eighty per cent, and the results showed that in only forty-eight per cent of deliveries did the same midwife attend throughout we would consider this a main finding.

In any study there may only be a small number of main findings, perhaps three or four. How easy was it to pick these out?

The results section of studies can look intimidating, especially if we do not have a full understanding of some of the statistical terminology and symbols. However, some of these meanings are easy to grasp (Clegg, 1982), and the results section can become clearer once we have learnt a few of the terms and symbols.

Although it is reasonable for authors to make some assumptions about the level of knowledge about statistical techniques, a reader has the right to feel that certain specialized terms and procedures should be clarified. If the author is interested in reaching the widest audience, then they should explain some of the terms. The author should also explain the tables, and graphs, so the reader can follow the reasoning being used to interpret the results. Understanding the results section can take time and perseverance. It is recommended that you refer to some of the more reader friendly books on statistics, such as the one by Clegg (1982).

In the end

The final part of the critique should look at the conclusion to the study, the recommendations, and then assess the way it has been presented and the implications for practice. Again, use the author's own words. Following the results of a study the author will present the issues that have arisen from the findings in the *'discussion'.* This section may also include the author's own comments on any limitations to the study, such as the sample, or the tool of data collection. These comments should be seen as positive, and part of research rigour, as the researcher is helping the reader to form a balanced view of the findings. The discussion section will then take some of the issues or implications raised by the results and put forward the author's interpretation of their relevance for an understanding of the topic. The literature may also be referred to again to underline the extent to which the findings in this particular study are similar to, or different from, those of other studies. While reading the discussion it is important to consider your own views of the arguments put forward. Do you agree, or are there other possible interpretations?

The final section of a research report should contain the *conclusion*, which provides an answer to the terms of reference. Although there may be a section headed 'conclusion', it may contain only recommendations, or broad statements that do not relate back to the terms of reference. The conclusion may be found in the discussion. Using some of the words from the terms of reference the conclusion should provide a succinct answer to the terms of reference, or say whether the hypotheses have been accepted or rejected. Where the terms of reference is made up of more than one part, question or hypothesis, each part should have a clear conclusion. In our assessment, we must consider whether the conclusion was based on, and supported by the results. Would we, given the findings of the study, have come to the same conclusions? Is the evidence strong enough to make that conclusion, or are there alternative conclusions which the author has not considered?

The final element may be the *recommendations*. What does the author suggest could improve the situation? Do these suggestions flow naturally from the discussion? One point to consider is whether the recommendations are realistic and concrete? Are they so vague and general that it is unlikely that improvements could be made? Do they give a clear idea of what it is the reader could go away and do, having read the report?

If we are to produce a critique of an article there are two remaining categories we need to consider. The first is how would we describe its *readability?* Although it can be argued that research convention dictates the way a study will be reported, and that it is this structure which can make research appear seem dull and uninteresting, we know from our own experience that this is not always so. Although we may be more interested in a study that touches on our particular area of work or own interests, any study has the potential to be presented in an interesting way.

We should expect that the writing is clear, with a minimum of jargon. Complex terminology should be explained or clarified as far as possible. It should be remembered, however, that the researcher may be entitled to feel that certain specialized terms are in common usage in research articles and that there is also an obligation on the reader to look up terms that may be unfamiliar to them, but which may be clear to the majority of readers of research.

Finally, we come to perhaps the most important section of all which is the *application to practice*. Once we have read it, what is the answer to the question 'so what?' We have to think about how the article as a whole may have a message for practice. Is there something that should now happen as a result of these findings? Perhaps we need to consider some of the points in the recommendations to see if there are some things that could relate to our own activities.

1. **Focus**
    In broad terms what is the theme of the article? What are the key words you would file this under? Is the title a clue to the focus? How important is this for the profession/practice?

2. **Background**
    What argument or evidence does the researcher provide which suggests this topic is worthwhile exploring? Is there a review of previous literature on the subject, or reference to government or professional reports that illustrate its importance? Are gaps in the literature or inadequacies with previous methods highlighted? Are local problems or changes that justify the study presented? Is there a trigger that answers the question 'why did they do it then?' Is there a theoretical or conceptual framework?

3. **Terms of reference**
    What is the aim of the research? This will usually start with the word 'to', e.g. the aim of this research was to examine/determine/compare/establish/ etc. If relevant, is there a hypothesis? If there is, what are the dependent and independent variables? Are there concept and operational definitions for the key concepts?

4. **Study design**
    What is the broad research approach? Is it experimental? Descriptive? Action research or audit? Is it quantitative or qualitative? Is the study design appropriate to the terms of reference?

5. **Data collection method**
    Which tool of data collection has been used? Has a single method been used or triangulation? Has the author addressed the issues of reliability and validity? Has a pilot study been conducted? Have any limitations of the tool been recognized by the author?

6. **Ethical considerations**
    Were the issues of informed consent, confidentiality, addressed? Was any harm or discomfort to individuals balanced against any benefits? Was the study considered by an ethics committee?

7. **Sample**
    Who or what makes up the sample? Are there clear inclusion and exclusion criteria? What method of sampling was used? Are those in the sample typical and representative, or are there any obvious elements of bias? On how many people/things/events are the results based?

8. **Data presentation**
    In what form are the results presented; tables, bar-graphs, pie-charts, raw figures, percentages? Does the author explain and comment on these? Has the author used correlation to establish whether certain variables are

associated with each other? Have tests of significance been used to establish to what extent any differences between groups/variables could have happened by chance? Can you make sense of the way the results have been presented, or could the author have provided more explanation?

9. **Main findings**
   Which are the most important results that relate to the terms of reference? (Think of this as putting the results in priority order; which is the most important result followed by the next most important result, etc. There may only be a small number of these.)

10. **Conclusion and recommendations**
    Using the author's own words, what is the answer to the terms of reference? If relevant, is the hypothesis accepted or rejected? Are the conclusions based on, and supported by the results? What recommendations are made for practice? Are these relevant, specific and feasible?

11. **Readability**
    How readable is it? Is it written in a clear, interesting, or 'heavy' style? Does it assume a lot of technical knowledge about the subject and/or research procedures (i.e. is there much jargon)?

12. **Practice implications**
    Once you have read it, what is the answer to the question 'so what?' Was it worth doing and publishing? How could it be related to practice? Who might find it relevant and in what way? What questions does it raise for practice and further study?

Box 4.1: Framework for critiquing quantitative research
(it is suggested that you photocopy this box, and use alongside relevant articles)

Once we have completed all the sections in Box 4.1, we should feel that we have a clear understanding of how the author carried out the study. We should also feel that we have not accepted the author's work uncritically. Critiquing a research article is a meeting of minds; ours and the researcher's. The result should be a greater understanding and consideration of the topic under study. It is emphasized that this should not automatically result in change; it may take other replication studies to produce a sufficient weight of evidence to suggest changes in practice. A single study, however, could make us question what we do, and its effectiveness. We might start to think whether some of our knowledge has passed its 'sell-by-date' and we need to look at our practices more critically.

If we have conducted the critique fairly, we should be able to evaluate research from a more informed, and objective standpoint, and not reject it simply because it does not agree with our own views on the subject. Midwifery needs its practitioners to exercise this skill for the benefit of all concerned. As a skill, though, it does need practice. As you work through this book you will gain more and more knowledge to apply when critiquing. It is immensely helpful if you can discuss your critique with others who have similar or more advanced skills in this. You should find that once you have used the framework for some time, you will begin to use it in your mind almost automatically, and you will not need to draw on the printed structure. You will then have reached the point where you have become an analytical consumer of research.

Critiquing qualitative research

The aim of qualitative research like that of quantitative research is to increase our knowledge, and so improve practice. As a number of areas important to midwifery do not lend themselves to numeric results and statistical accuracy, other methodological approaches are applicable. Qualitative research is one such alternative.

There are a number of different categories of qualitative research, but Holloway and Wheeler (1996) suggest that they have the following basic principles in common:

- They take the point of view of the subjects of the research. This is called 'the insiders' or 'emic' perspective.
- Researchers immerse themselves in the setting and involve themselves with the subjects and the culture to which they belong.
- Data are not collected according to a predetermined theoretical framework, but the reverse; the data are used to develop a theory.
- The researcher provides 'thick' description of the way the study was undertaken, this describes what took place in the study in sufficient depth for the reader to almost experience for themselves what it was like in that setting.
- The relationship between the researcher and those in the study is close and is one of equality and respect.
- Analysis takes place at the same time as data collection.

These features emphasize the differences in the way the research is conducted and presented and illustrate why the use of the critiquing framework presented in the previous section is not just difficult, but in many ways inappropriate. Any attempt to use the quantitative approach to critiquing would inevitably lead to unfair criticism, as the way qualitative research is conducted appears to break many of the principles of quantitative research. These includes such things as establishing 'scientific' (i.e. measurable) objectivity and the maintenance of social distance between the researcher and those involved in the study to avoid bias and 'contaminating' the results. From a midwifery point of view, however, this approach, which concentrates on understanding and insight, seems eminently suitable and compatible with a woman centred focus of care.

Although qualitative research is similar to quantitative research in its desire to be accurate and rigorous, we need to adapt the critiquing framework to take account of the different principles and philosophy of the approach. In this section some of the essential features of qualitative research are outlined and are related to a framework for critiquing qualitative reports (see Box 4.2).

Focus and background

Qualitative research identifies a particular problem which needs exploring and this centres on a key concept, issue or theme. Morse and Field (1996) have noted that whether the research is quantitative or qualitative, it must be worth the effort. The researcher should, therefore, provide a clear rationale as to why the study has been undertaken. This will consist of the identification of important professional issues, local details, or key concepts relevant to the profession or clinical practice. These key concepts should be clearly defined in the background to the study. In the case of some forms of qualitative research, such as grounded theory, the researcher avoids reading too much literature prior to data collection. This is in case it influences the way the data is collected and prejudges what are deemed to be important issues. In preference, the researcher will allow respondents to define the important issues. Other forms of qualitative research may present a critical review of the literature, in the same way as quantitative studies. The researcher will state a terms of reference, but this may be deliberately broad to provide flexibility and avoid preconceived ideas. It may well simply say the intention is to examine the experience, or perception of some concept or other.

Methodology

In outlining the methodology, the researcher should be as rigorous as the quantitative researcher, and illustrate the steps taken to make the process of data collection as accurate as possible. As an attempt is made to avoid separating subjects from the social contexts in which they function, there should be rich or 'thick' descriptions of the setting. Talbot (1995) defines 'thick' description as 'description that enumerates everything that another would need to know to comprehend the researcher's conclusions'. This should be so detailed that we almost feel ourselves to be there.

As the researcher attempts to be as flexible as possible in collecting the data and will attempt to analyse the data along with data collection, there will rarely be a pilot study. This brings into question the issue of the reliability of the data collection tool. Whereas the quantitative researcher is influenced by reliability and validity, according to LoBiondo-Wood and Haber (1995) the concerns of the qualitative researcher are *credibility, auditability* and *fittingness*. Credibility relates to the extent to which the researcher tries to ensure the accuracy of the results, auditability relates to the extent to which the researcher provides details on how categories were developed from the data collected, and fittingness relates to the extent to which the results are applicable outside the specific context in which the study was undertaken.

The sample size of qualitative research tends to be much smaller than quantitative research as data collection is a more lengthy process. The aim is not to produce a sample that is statistically similar to the larger population; the intention is to included those in a position to talk in an informed way about the concept of concern to the study. In qualitative research the researcher is often dependent on 'informants' who volunteer information, or agree to provide an insider's view of things. We should expect, however, that there is an attempt to acknowledge and limit bias as much as possible so that the range of experiences or opinions is covered by the sample. Once the researcher feels that subjects are repeating what has previously been revealed, they may end data collection on the grounds that 'saturation' has been reached, and further respondents would not add anything new to the study. Morse and Field (1996) suggest that the researcher should ensure the sample size is large enough to exclude those who were not good informants, or from whom nothing was learned.

The issues of ethics should also be addressed as they are just as important in this type of research as in any other. Here the researcher attempts to ensure that the individual is not put at any disadvantage as a result of being part of the study and should gain informed consent from respondents. Where appropriate the Local Research Ethics Committee (LREC) will also be approached to give approval for the study. American studies will refer to an Institutional Review Boards (IRB) which serves the same purpose.

Analysis

It is true to say that the crucial part of qualitative research is the analysis. At this point the researcher inductively analyses the findings for what they might reveal about the subject of the study. If the researcher is to avoid the accusation of subjectivity, they should make it clear how decisions have been made throughout the research so that the reader can understand the thinking employed, not only in conducting the research, but also in the analysis of the findings. This should take the form of a 'decision trail' for the reader to follow.

The results section of qualitative research is frequently referred to as the 'findings', and differs from that of quantitative research as it will take the form of quotes, either from a respondent, or dialogue involving both a respondent and the researcher. It may also include descriptions of places, or events, some of these will be extracts from the researcher's 'fieldwork diary' or notebook.

Morse and Field (1996) warn that it is not enough to simply present dialogue or quotes in the findings section, as the researcher must be more than the editor of an audio taped story. They suggest that the comments surrounding quotations in the text should be thoughtfully re discussed and brought to a general level of discussion and not left to 'speak for itself'. Along with the presentation of this form of data, the findings section may also include reference to the literature which is used as part of establishing credibility for the results of the study, as well as contributing to the analysis of the data.

Conclusion

The conclusion of the study may not only include the answer to the terms of reference, but may also put forward a possible hypothesis regarding the focus of the study and suggest some relationship to other variables. This may also result in the statement of a theory, or a conceptual framework that may be explored through subsequent research.

Application to practice

The reader of qualitative research will want to draw out the relevance of the research for practice, and the profession as a whole. As one of the aims of qualitative research is to sensitize the reader to the position of those in the study, the application to practice will include the extent to which new insights and awareness have been achieved through reading the study. Although it is often assumed that the findings of qualitative research are not generalizable, Morse and Field (1996) make the point that it is the theory and insights established by the study that are applicable to other situations. The rigour relating to the way in which the research has been conducted will also be brought into question at this point, as the accuracy of the findings must be considered, and the extent to which any theoretical or conceptual frameworks really do fit the situation described.

This outline of the framework for qualitative research indicates that this form of research is no less rigorous than other forms. The way in which the reader approaches the published work is no less systematic than any other study. Although the research can appear very descriptive it can be as beneficial to practice as experimental research. This is because it can provide insights into practice and experiences that may not be possible for the individual midwife to access and so provide a more informed and sensitive approach to care.

1. **Focus**

   What is the key issue, concept or problem that this work examines? What are the key words you would file this under? Are there clues to the focus in title? How important is this for practice and the profession?

2. **Background**

   What argument or evidence does the researcher provide for exploring this issue, concept or problem? Is there a review of previous literature on the subject or reference to government or professional reports that illustrate its importance? Are gaps in the literature or inadequacies with previous methods highlighted? Does the literature review examine the concepts or issues that form the focus? Is there an attempt to justify the study within the context of a qualitative research design? If this is grounded theory there may not be a comprehensive review of the literature at this point, although some reference to previous work may be presented as an illustration of its importance. There should be some argument or background information to justify looking at this particular subject.

3. **Terms of reference**

   What is the stated aim of the research? This will usually start with the word 'to...'. There will not be a hypothesis or the identification of dependent and independent variables, as qualitative research is usually a level 1 question. There may be an attempt to provide a concept definition for the concept that forms the focus of the study.

4. **Study design**

   There may an acknowledgement that the study is qualitative and then a statement made on the specific approach that has been used. The main alternatives are i) *phenomenological*, which explores what it is like to have a certain experience such as a delivery, a pregnancy or threatened miscarriage, and how people interpret that experience; ii) *ethnographic*, where the researcher enters and participates in the world of the subject by listening, observing and asking questions in order to understand their view of the world, or iii) *grounded theory*, which will identify concepts which arise from the analysis of the data collected, and may also suggest a theory or hypothesis which explains or predicts relationships between some of the concepts which have emerged in the study. It is important that the philosophy behind the method suits the intentions of the research.

5. **Tool of data collection**

   Here we are interested not only in the technique used to collect the information, but the amount of detail we have on the circumstances under which the data were collected. This contributes to the *credibility* of the study. This should include details of the environment in which the data were collected, over what period of time data collection took place, and any other details that allow us to visualize the conduct of data collection. Did the researcher spend sufficient time, either in observing the life and behaviour of the subjects, or in interviewing subjects, to produce sufficient depth to the data? Because of the flexible way that data are gathered, and the way the method will change during data collection, a pilot study will not usually be employed. The researcher should, however, include detail of how they have attempted to achieve *procedural rigour* in the way the study was conducted. Did they check with those in the study that the information collected was accurate (member's check)?

6. **Ethical considerations**

   As with qualitative studies, it is important that the researcher has protected the respondent from harm, and has gained informed consent from those taking part in the study. It should not be possible to identify individuals or places where the study took place. The researcher should illustrate ethical rigour, including where appropriate approaching a Local Research Ethics Committee (LREC), or in American studies an Institutional Review Board (IRB), to approve the research.

7. **Sample**

   Who makes up the sample and what are their basic characteristics? The sample size may be quite small, and dictated by theoretical saturation, that is data collection stops once there is a repetition in the type of information or categories being revealed. In qualitative research it is important to assess whether the respondents or subjects possess the relevant knowledge or carry out the activity in which the researcher is interested. Has the researcher demonstrated that the subjects are able to provide relevant information and are not open to any kind of bias? The reader must consider to what extent the findings, theory or conceptual categories may apply to other settings. This contributes to its *fittingness* to be applied elsewhere.

8. **Data presentation**

   The data will be presented in the form of description, dialogue or comments from respondents. Is this 'thick' and 'rich' description? Is there sufficient detail for us to almost feel that we are there? Do the quotes from respondents clearly illustrate the concepts they are being used to illustrate? Is there over-dependence on comments from a small number of the respondents in the sample? Has the researcher detailed how they ensured that the data were accurately recorded and representative of the data gathered? Is there anything about the circumstances in which the data were collected that could have threatened the accuracy of the data? Is it possible to discover the 'decision trail' used by the researcher to determine how the raw data was processed into the categories presented in the results section? This contributes to its *auditability.* Given the same data it should be possible following the decision trail to arrive at similar categories and results. Does the researcher present the findings in the subjects own words rather than reinterpreting what was said or done?

9. **Main findings**

   What are the key concepts or categories developed from the data? Do the concepts and categories presented cover all the data gathered? Were the findings checked either by the respondents (members check) or examined by other experts in the field? Are the main findings *credible*, that is, have attempts been made to support the accuracy of the results through rigour in the way in which the study was conducted? Does the researcher discuss the findings and relate these to the literature, or do they appear to believe that the quotes will speak for themselves?

10. **Conclusion**

    Is there a clear answer to the terms of reference? Does the researcher propose a relationship between the concepts and categories developed in the analysis to form a clear conceptual or theoretical framework? Does the conceptual or theoretical framework reflect the data? Has the conclusion been arrived at inductively on the basis of the findings?

11. **Readability**

    Does the researcher present the description of the social circumstances described in the research in sufficient detail that one can almost imagine being there, and hear the respondents talking and carrying out the activities described? Is it possible to recognize the concepts described as related to practical experience? Is the way the report is written clear and understandable? Is there a clear 'story line' emerging from the research?

12. Relevance to practice
Are the findings relevant to practice or professional knowledge? Is it an important area related to current concerns and issues within the profession? Does the research satisfy the criteria of transferability, that is, can the findings in the form of the theory, concepts or categories developed through the study be applied to other situations, or are they only applicable to the place and the people where the study took place? Do you feel the research has sensitized you to issues or provided further insight? Has it confirmed views you might have already held?

Box 4.2: Framework for critiquing qualitative research
(it is suggested that you photocopy this box, and use alongside relevant articles)

Conducting research

There are two reasons why this chapter is relevant to those undertaking research. Firstly, the skill of critiquing is an essential part of reviewing the literature, and therefore the researcher should approach the literature in a critical and analytical way. The methods outlined here are therefore important for the researcher to apply when considering the work of others.

Secondly, the researcher should remember that at the conclusion of their study a report will be written, and perhaps an article published. These will be subjected to the type of scrutiny suggested here. If the researcher is aware of the criteria and framework the reader will use to evaluate their work, then they can ensure that these areas are addressed when communicating the study.

In this section on qualitative research, it has been emphasized how important it is for the researcher to paint a very clear and vivid picture of their experience in conducting the study. This process is facilitated through the use of a field work diary, or field-notes (Morse and Field, 1996). These should contain all the essential descriptive elements relating to the field work. In the same way they should also contain the major analytical processes that unfolded throughout data analysis. It is from these that the researcher can clearly describe their decision trail and illuminates how the different conceptual categories arose from the mass of findings.

Critiquing research

This chapter has emphasized the need to question and critically analyse published research. If practice is to be evidence based it is necessary to develop analytical skills. This should not be a purely negative activity, but should take a balanced view identifying both strengths and weaknesses. Remember, research is a difficult activity and it is important to identify the limitations of a study whilst recognizing the constraints under which research is conducted.

Critiquing is a skill, and as such requires practice. It is useful if discussion on research articles takes place between practitioners. These can be on an informal basis, or on a more formal level, as in the case of journal clubs, and research interest groups. In either context it is important to be systematic in the way the critique is conducted. It is also important that the appropriate critiquing format has been used on the research. There is no use applying the quantitative critiquing framework, on a qualitative article. This chapter has attempted to provide a suitable framework in order for you to critique articles, and research reports. You might find it useful to photocopy the two tables so that you have a more readily accessible check list to follow when critiquing.

KEY POINTS

- The researcher rarely has the ideal conditions under which to conduct research, and so weakness can be found in most published research. Just because a piece of research has been published does not mean it is above constructive criticism.

- In order to critique an article it is important to use a systematic approach. This chapter has provided two critique frameworks; one that can applied to quantitative research articles, and one that can be applied to qualitative research. As quantitative research is based on completely different principles from those of qualitative, it is important that the criteria for judging one are not applied to the other.

- A critique should have a balance between description – what the researcher(s) did, and analysis – how well has it been done? It is not a negative criticism of a piece of research, but should recognize strengths, as well as limitations. Undertaking a critique provides a sound basis for establishing research based practice, as it ensures that published research is carefully evaluated and not accepted on face value.

CHAPTER FIVE

Reviewing the Literature

A review of the literature can be defined as the critical examination of a representative selection of published literature on a particular topic or issue. This is carried out for three main reasons. Firstly, it is part of the research process where the aim is to inform the researcher on the present state of knowledge on the topic covered by the study. It also provides the researcher with valuable information on the methods used in previous studies which might influence the present approach. Secondly, a review of the literature is an important end in itself in the clinical area, and can provide a balanced view on the current state of knowledge on a topic that might influence practice. It can also be used to provide the basis for clinical protocols, or audit standards. Finally, a review of the literature is a frequent activity within many courses of study, either as an important element within an assignment, or as the main focus of an assignment.

The purpose of a review can be seen from the following list suggested by LoBiondo-Wood and Haber (1994):

1. Determines what is known and not known about a subject, concept or problem.
2. Determines gaps, consistencies and inconsistencies in the literature concerning a subject, concept or problem.
3. Discovers unanswered questions about a subject, concept or problem.
4. Describes the strengths and weaknesses of designs or methods of inquiry and instruments used in earlier research.
5. Discovers conceptual traditions used to examine problems.
6. Generates useful research questions, projects or activities for the discipline.
7. Determines an appropriate research design or method (instruments, data collection and analysis methods) for answering research questions.
8. Determines the need for replication of a well-designed study or refinement of a study.
9. Promotes development of protocols and policies related to clinical practice.
10. Uncovers developments in practice intervention, or gains support for changing a practice intervention.

The purpose of this chapter is to provide practical advice on undertaking a critical review of the literature. As with research activity, there is a clear process that can be followed, and this consists of the following three broad stages, each with its own demands and skills required to accomplish them:

- locating the literature;
- extracting relevant detail;
- writing the review.

There are clear parallels between a review of the literature and a research project. They both start with a clear question, and maximum effort must go into the planning stage. It is no use saying, 'I want to find out about women who have twins'. To be successful, you have to be clear on why you are carrying out the review, and think what questions you want the review to answer. It would be far better to have a question such as what are the main physical, psychological and social problems faced by women who have twins? If you are carrying out the review as part of the research process, you will also want to establish, 'what are the most successful ways of answering this question?'

The aim of the review should be specific, and may consist of a number of subheadings under which you will group the literature. The usual headings, which concentrate on content, are listed in Box 5.1.

- What (definitions)
- Why (what are the causes/influences)
- Who (is particularly affected/at risk/involved)
- When (are there particular times when this might happen or action should be taken)
- How (does it happen/take place/can we do something about it)
- Advantages
- Disadvantages
- Problems
- Solutions/recommendations.

Box 5.1: Theme headings for structuring a review

Not all of these would be used for every subject. If we take an example we can see how they can be applied in practice (see Box 5.2).

Aim of the review:
To consider the implications of twins on the mother and family in terms of physical, psychological and social factors, and to identify the implications for the midwife.

Possible theme headings:

- What are twins – how is this clinically defined, what variations are there?
- Why do twins occur – what are the factors associated with twin pregnancies?
- Who is most likely to have twins?

- When should some of the implications be considered?
- How do twins influence physical, psychological, social factors related to the mother and family?
- Problems – what problems are associated with twins in pregnancy, delivery, and early months?
- Solutions – how can some of the identified problems be reduced?
- What are the implications for the midwife?

If at this stage it is clear that the resultant review is going to be large, it can be decided to look at an aspect of it, such as looking at the consequence of twins in the first six months following delivery. In this way the planning stage helps to clarify the question the review will answer. It is also important to realize that some of the above questions will have a different emphasis in terms of how much space will be devoted to the topic. Some will be discussed in a sentence or two, others will be several pages long.

Box 5.2: Planning a review of the literature

Finding the literature

We are now in a position to think about finding the literature. The first location which springs to mind is a library. Nowadays most health libraries of any size, particularly if they have an educational function, have a CD Rom. This is a computer which holds details of published articles on a wide variety of topics. These require a key word, or key words to be typed in, before it is able to provide a list of articles with those words in the title, or summary of the article. The problem is frequently finding the right word under which appropriate articles are stored. So for instance 'parentcraft' may not work but 'antenatal education' might.

Once the CD Rom has identified some likely titles, it is a case of locating them. This is where the problems frequently begin. The list of articles may include many references to articles in journals not stocked by the library. Although it is sometimes possible to order them through inter-library loan, this is costly. Some libraries can be reluctant to supply above a certain number, so it is worth ensuring that they are likely to be essential to your review before ordering. Where the library does stock the journal there can still be a number of problems, these include:

- the library not having the journal for that time period;
- all the copies being there apart from the one you want;
- the library appearing to keep it, but a complete search of the shelves, and the desks failing to locate it;
- the copy being there, but the pages you want are missing.

For these reasons it is important to avoid depending solely on this source of information in the library. Sapsford and Abbott (1992) suggest that of all the resources in a library, the most important is the librarian. Although many people may feel that this does not correspond to their experience, it is important to use the potential of the staff. They are there to help you, providing that your requests are reasonable. They will rarely, for instance, carry out a search for you, but they will help you understand how to carry out the search yourself.

Sapsford and Abbott (1992) suggest that using a system such as the CD Rom may be the 'approved' way of locating references, but it is not always the most productive and suggest the following alternatives for finding relevant books and articles.

1. Identify the catalogue reference that most closely fits the topic you are searching for and just look along the shelves at this point to see what the library has in stock.

2. Look through the issues covering the last couple of years of relevant journals.

3. Starting from articles you have been able to find, look at their reference lists to identify other articles or books which may be relevant.

The last suggestion can be called 'backward chaining' where the reviewer goes back by following the chain of references from article to article. Whatever method is chosen, the words of Brink and Wood (1994) are very true when they say that 'the actual mechanics of a literature review requires legwork on your part'. At the end of this phase of the process you should have a reasonable number of references on which to base your review.

Extracting relevant details

Once you have located material, the next step is to extract relevant information for your review. Many people achieve this stage with the help of a fluorescent highlighter pen. This can be a problem though when you are left with very few lines on a page which do not have a bright yellow, pink or green line through it. When it comes to writing the review, this is not a useful way of identifying appropriate quotes as they are difficult to locate.

What are the alternatives to the highlighter pen? Gould (1995) suggests the use of index cards on which are written a journal or book title. These should be written in the approved referencing system you are using, or that recommended by the course or institute to which you belong. These cards should be kept in the correct system (either in alphabetical order or the sequence in which they occur in the text). Relevant details and comments can then be added to the card which covers some of the key points.

A better system is to have not only a set of cards containing the details of each author, but a second set on which are written the quotes you would usually have highlighted with a pen. These 'quote cards' should also have the name of the author and year of publication to cross-reference with the author cards. They should also include the page number so the quote can be relocated, and the theme under which the quote will be filed. It is important to think of the review as being structured under various theme headings. A review is frequently built around the answers to the questions posed in Box 5.1.

Cards relating to similar themes can then be kept together. When it comes to the writing stage, the cards can be spread out so you can clearly see the information gathered. Those points that are similar can then be discussed together, and the sequence of points planned out before the writing begins. This is a lot easier than having information underlined throughout the numerous photocopies you may have, and be faced with the difficulty of trying to remember what information was where?

An alternative to index cards is the use of a critique 'grid'. This consists of a large sheet of paper, such as flip chart paper, or even the back of a sheet of wallpaper, divided into columns. Each column should contain one of the theme headings. Where an article is a piece of research the following columns will also be useful to act as a summary and which will then allow comparisons to be made between different research articles:

- Terms of reference/hypothesis
- Research design/method of data collection
- Sample size and inclusion and exclusion criteria
- Main results (briefly)
- Conclusion
- Recommendations
- Strengths and limitations of the study.

As with the card system, when reading an article or book, it is possible to skim, or speed-read until material relevant to one of the headings in the grid is encountered. The material is then read slowly and a decision made as to whether some or all of this should be entered in the grid.

Once an article has been exhausted, a line is ruled across the page and a new article examined. As with the cards, it is worth adding the page number following each extract so that it can be relocated if necessary, and can be quoted exactly with the page number if required. Material relevant to each column will not necessarily appear in each paper, so some columns may be blank for some authors. The advantage of this method is that all material relating to the same theme can be read by looking up and down a column and analysed for a pattern of similarities or differences between authors.

A final method relates to the use of a personal computer. If you normally produce your written work directly on a word processing programme, the following system will save a lot of time. Instead of using a grid, create a number of files and name each one according to the themes you have decided to use in your review. As you work your way through each source of information, you can open the appropriate file, and type in the comments you wish to record. Start each quote with the name of the author, the year of publication and page number. Time can be reduced on a number of word processors if you highlight the author's name, and year of publication, and 'copy'. This will then be placed on the computers' 'clipboard'. Each time you add another quote from the same source, use the 'paste' function. The author's name and year of publication will appear ready for you to add the page number and the quote you want to record. You can continue to paste in the name and year for each additional entry, providing nothing further has been copied as this will 'over-write' what is on the clipboard. If you use this word processing system you may want to print out a hard copy to check the material visually. You can also reorder the material if you so wish.

Common questions

At this stage there are usually a number of questions you may have concerning the review. One of the most frequent question asked by students is 'how many articles do I need for my review?' There is no magic number. The advice is to get hold of as many articles as you can in as short a period of time as possible. The more articles you gather, the easier it will be to see a pattern. If time is limited, there should be two main priority areas, and they are to include as much recent material as possible, as these will contain current thinking and evidence, and secondly, include as many of the 'classics' as possible. The latter are the titles that seem to crop up in the majority of writers work on a particular topic.

A second question is how far back do I need to go? The usual method is to go back three or five years. If there is a lot of material, it may be relevant to make the time period shorter, if there is very little material, it may be beneficial to go back further.

A further question is do all the articles have to be research articles? The answer to this is that it is acceptable to include some descriptive reports based on individual thoughts, opinions or experiences, but where possible concentrate on research articles as they are the result of a more systematic process.

A final question relates to the use of primary and secondary sources. A primary source is the original work of an author, a secondary source is where someone has quoted, or examined the work of another author. Where it is not possible to get hold of the original work quickly, it is tempting to use secondary sources. These can appear useful where they include critical comment on the primary work. However, there is general agreement that these sources should not be overused, and that where possible the primary source should be consulted (LoBiondo-Wood and Haber, 1994).

Writing the review

Producing the written review is a high level skill. It is not simply a collection of quotes 'cut out' of the literature, nor is it a series of critiques of individual research articles. It should contain both description of the literature with analysis and reflection on what the literature contains, how well it is presented, and how it all relates to the question the review is seeking to answer. The approach used in writing the review is brought out in the following observation from Benton and Cormack (1996):

> 'A review of the literature should be written objectively with all criticism being based on factual material and supported by appropriate evidence and argument. In addition, any review should be balanced with both the positive and negative aspects of material being discussed. Furthermore the implications of any flaws identified in previous work must be highlighted. A good literature review will provide far more than the critical appraisal of a series of articles, it should create a structure upon which further research can be based.'

This gives clear guidelines to follow in using the material gathered. But how can we judge the quality of the review in terms of its usefulness? Again Benton and Cormack (1996) make the following suggestion:

> 'Unless the literature is analysed in detail and the interrelationships between previous publications identified, the quality of the review will be poor. Inadequate analysis and synthesis of literature results in a review that may only present a series of disjointed paragraphs that echo the findings of previous studies. By planning the review, a logical, structured and coherent argument for further research, or an appraisal of the current state of our knowledge can be presented.'

The point made here is to avoid the temptation to include as many references as possible, simply because they have been found. They must make sense within the review. The number of references used is much less important than the relevance of the references, the quality of the comments and the overall organization. In the end it must answer the question that has been stated as the aim of the review, and end by saying what we can now say about the topic based on the literature, in particular what is the relevance to practice, or midwifery knowledge.

At this stage it is possible to suggest a review of the literature process which should be followed which takes account of all three sections covered so far. This process is presented in Box 5.3 below.

---

1. Decide on a clear question you want to answer through the review.

2. Plan the structure of the review by thinking of the themes that will be applicable. Remember that the following are useful starting points; what, why, when, who, how, advantages and disadvantages or problems and solutions.

3. Decide on the key words you may need for the topic.

4. Identify possible sources of locating references, and actual literature. Explore a library armed with your key words, consult a data base such as MIDIRS, or the Cochrane data base. Don't forget to be creative, and use backward chaining if you find articles look at their references, use colleagues, other students, people in education, and specialists in the topic.

5. If there seems too little material, broaden the topic, if there is too much focus the topic down to one aspect.

6. Decide on a time period to be covered. Initially this could be five years. If there is too little, go back further, if there is too much reduce the number of years. Remember it might be wise to include the classics in the field.

7. As you locate material, whether it is articles, books or reports, ensure that all the information for a complete reference is written on an author card.

---

8. Read through the material with your theme headings in mind. Scan fast until you meet with relevant material and then slow down and decide whether to extract it.

9. Enter the important material onto cards, a grid, or onto your computer file. Don't forget your own comments on the material.

10. Examine your material for patterns by comparing and contrasting different authors.

11. Write a rough draft under the theme headings. Make sure you have both description (what the various authors say) as well as analysis (how well they say it). Make connections between the material for your reader, and don't forget the purpose of the review. Keep telling the reader why the material included is relevant.

12. When you are ready for the main draft, write a clear introduction, which includes the purpose of the review, the parameters used to select the material (the source of the material, e.g. British and American, and the time period it covers), and the themes which have been used to group the literature.

13. At the end make sure you relate the literature to practice. What can we say now based on the literature. The conclusion should comment not only on the subject and what has been learnt, but on the literature itself. Is the available literature comprehensive, or are there gaps? Is the research carried out on the subject of a high standard and rigorous, or does it contain weaknesses?

14. Remember, a review is not an essay that puts forward your views supported selectively by the literature. Neither is it a series of critiques. In writing the review, you should always start from the literature, what does it say?

Box 5.3: The process of reviewing the literature

Conducting research

A thorough review of the literature increases the researcher's ability to plan research effectively and efficiently. So much can be learned from the published work of others, both in terms of content – what has already been established, and process – how have others gone about exploring this topic. It is important that the review is comprehensive. The researcher should take advantage of as many sources of information as possible. There should be an emphasis on more recent material as this may provide information about more recent findings, understanding and new approaches. Classic pieces of literature and reports should also be included.

The researcher should consider the literature critically, and compare and contrast the views and findings of authors. This should be considered in the light of the intended project. In particular, examine concept and operational definitions, and details of data collect tools. The method of data analysis and presentation should also be considered for the way in which they might be a model for the present study.

Critiquing research

When critiquing a research article, the review of the literature section can provide a lot of information on what stimulated the thinking of the researcher. The design and the nature of the research question will have been influenced by what the researcher discovered in their review. This should be clearly communicated in the report.

Some of the preliminary pointers the reader should consider include the extent of the review – how much literature is included, and how up-to-date is it? Are there any pieces of work obviously missing? In particular, the reader should consider the extent to which the writer critically reviews the available literature. Do they identify weakness, and gaps in the literature that will be addressed in their study?

The review of the literature should inform the reader and provide a clear rationale for conducting the study. Reading the review should provide an understanding of some of the key issues related to the topic and should also indicate some of the research that has already been undertaken and which forms a backdrop to the current study. In some cases the review will also support the theoretical or conceptual framework which has been used in a study. This will link the key concepts together to show how they are seen to be related to each other.

KEY POINTS

- A review of the literature is a critical analysis of the pertinent published work on a topic.

- Carrying out a review has a great deal to offer individual midwives and clinical areas in increasing the standard of evidence based practice.

- Reviewing the literature is a skill that can be developed through the application of the principles outlined in this chapter.

- Finding the literature is influenced firstly by the identification of the relevant key words under which the literature may be accessed.

- A well-stocked library is essential, but there are a number of other systems available that will also prove useful, such as the use of MIDIRS. It is important to be systematic in the method used to retrieve information from individual books and articles. This chapter has provided several examples.

- In writing the review the topic should be presented under relevant themes; a review is not a series of critiques joined together.

- To be relevant to practice the review should be written to include description and critical analysis.

CHAPTER SIX

The Research Question

One of the crucial stages of the research process is the development of the research question. It is on this stage that so many other parts of the research process depend. But where do research questions come from and what makes a good research question? This chapter will outline the importance of the research question, and answer these important questions. The construction of a hypothesis will also be examined, and the type of research that requires a hypothesis will be outlined.

The importance of the research question

If we compare research to setting out on a journey, then the research question is the statement of the destination. We cannot map a clear and effective route unless we know where we are going, and we certainly will not know whether we have arrived, unless we know where we want to be at the end of the journey. In the same way, the research question allows the researcher to plan the research in the best possible way, and make important decisions to ensure that the correct destination is reached.

The following are the main elements in the research process which will be influenced by the research question:

- the broad research approach (methodology);
- the tool of data collection (the method);
- the sample;
- the form of data analysis;
- the ethical considerations.

We can see what Cormack and Benton (1996) meant when they said:

'Unless you have a clearly defined research question you will be unable to progress your study in a planned and efficient manner. You cannot undertake a research study without identifying a research question.'

According to Rees (1995b), midwifery is full of questions that need answers. The research question is developed from a broad topic area which the researcher has decided to explore. Where does the topic come from? Some are prompted by service problems, or a desire to improve the quality of the service offered, others arise from reviewing the literature, or from establishing ways to achieve government directives such as 'Changing Childbirth' (DoH, 1993).

Can research be carried out to answer every midwifery question? It depends. Some questions demand a value judgement for their solution, and are not open to research. For example, should midwives carry out more of the technological procedures currently carried out by obstetricians? Although we can survey midwives' views or those of obstetricians, the answers would not indicate whether it is 'right', only what people feel about it. Similarly, some questions are ethical or philosophical questions and cannot be answered by research but need to be discussed and debated.

One important issue to consider before pursuing a research question is that of relevance. Does the research need to be done? Every project should be evaluated in terms of the contribution it will make to midwifery. This may be in terms of increasing knowledge, or practice, developing or testing midwifery theory, or helping to shape policy. Cormack and Benton (1996) further develop the issue of relevance and suggest the following criteria:

> 'First does the question address a problem which affects a large number of (people)? Second, will the outcome of the research significantly improve the quality of life of individuals or groups? Third, does the question address a (midwifery) problem? Finally, will the results be suitable for use in a (non-research) practice environment?'

Perhaps one of the most important criteria to consider when judging the relevance of a research project is will women, their babies and the family unit benefit? Even if the topic relates to midwives themselves, those receiving care may still benefit indirectly through an increase or change in midwives' knowledge, skills or attitudes.

The final point made by Cormack and Benton above is also important, in that unless it is possible to introduce the change into midwifery practice, and overcome the barriers of cost, lack of training or skills, and particularly resistance to change, the research will be a wasted effort.

Following a consideration of the relevance of research, the next major issue is feasibility. This includes such factors as the time available, researcher expertise, ethical consideration, resources available, subject availability and the co-operation of others.

The type of question

The research question is important because of the consequences it has for many of the other elements in the research process. The form the question takes will suggest the level of the question as categorized by Brink and Wood (1994). Some of the questions midwifery research attempts to answer are shown in Box 6.1. The way the question is posed or 'framed' will illustrate the level it addresses. This is important as it influences the broad research approach. A level 1 question will suggest the use of a survey or a qualitative approach such as an ethnographic or phenomenological study. A level 2 question may also suggest a survey, but the question will mention more than one variable. This level may also include the collection of physiological measurements through observation or taking samples where at least two different measures from each subject are compared statistically to see if they show a similar pattern or correlation. A level 3 question is one that suggests that comparisons may be made between two variables in order to see if they are different, or that a particular theory or hypothesis is being tested.

The question may also imply a likely methods of data collection. Although in many cases a choice may exist, such as between the use of questionnaire and interviews, some questions will suggest the more appropriate method. A level 3 question will usually make it clear that a form of experimental design will be needed.

The question will also suggest the type of data to be collected. In the main this will relate to whether quantitative data will be gathered, in the form of numbers, or whether qualitative data in the form of words will be necessary. This in turn will have implications for the type of statistic that will be appropriate to use (see Box 6.1).

QUESTION	APPROACH	METHOD	DATA	STATISTIC
what are we/they doing? how well are we/they doing it? what do people think? (level 1)	descriptive survey audit	observation questionnaires interviews documents	quantitative in the form of numbers	descriptive, frequency averages, ranges, standard deviation
what is it like? how does it feel? how do people behave? (level 1)	descriptive ethnographic phenomenological	in depth interviews, sustained observation, documentary accounts (personal diaries, etc.)	words in the form of dialogue, extracts of observed situations conversations	rarely appropriate apart from frequency tables
what is related to, or associated with, what? (level 2)	correlational survey, physiological measurement	questionnaires interviews observation documents	quantitative in the form of numbers	inferential in the form of correlation
is this way better/more effective than that? (level 2/3) is there evidence to demonstrate that the theory can be used to predict outcome (level 3)	quasi-experimental, experimental (randomized control trials)	physiological measurements, questionnaires interviews frequent use of scales e.g. visual analogue scales for pain etc.	quantitative in the form of numbers	inferential in the form of tests of significance

Box 6.1: Examples of different research questions

Constructing a research question

How do we construct a research question? Cormack and Benton (1996) point out that research questions can occur in one of two forms, one is the *interrogative* and the other is the *declarative*. The interrogative form is structured in exactly the same way as a question. For example, 'what influences women to continue breastfeeding further than four weeks?' The second form, the declarative statement, is used more often in research reports, and is a statement of the purpose of the study. This identifies what particular event, phenomenon or situation the study is going to consider and usually starts with such words as:

> 'to examine'
> 'to identify'
> 'to describe'
> 'to explore'

An example would be 'to identify some of the factors which influence a women to breastfeed further than four weeks'.

In Chapter 2 we defined this way of expressing the research question as the *terms of reference* of a study. In other words, this is the statement the researcher 'refers to' in designing the study. The statement of the terms of reference should allow the reader to identify what will happen to whom. This means there should be an indication of what information is to be gathered, or what variable is being examined, perhaps in relation to another variable, and from whom or what this information will be collected. Box 6.2 illustrates some examples of terms of reference written in this style.

When constructing a research question an easy way to develop the terms of reference is to say 'what is the purpose of my study?' The answer, starting with the word 'to ... ', will form the terms of reference.

AUTHOR	TERMS OF REFERENCE	LEVEL
Hughes and Rees (1997)	to establish what influences women to bottle feed	1
Floyd (1995)	to investigate how midwives feel about undertaking home births and to explore the factors influencing their beliefs	1
Paterson et al. (1994)	to assess the effect of low haemoglobin on the mental and physical health of postnatal women	2
Bannon (1994)	to determine the effect of amniotomy on labour and neonatal outcome	3

Box 6.2: Examples of terms of reference

At this point it is worth recalling the different levels of research questions, suggested by Brink and Wood (1994), as it will enable us to consider the elements we would expect to find at each level. In Chapter 2 we saw that level one questions are those where little is known about a topic and the intention is to describe a situation. There is only one variable in a level 1 question and one population to which it belongs. The researcher should give a clear concept definition which relates to the way the variable will be defined for the purposes of the study. There should also be an operational definition which will outline the way it is intended to measure that variable. At this level there is no attempt to establish cause and effect relationships between variables.

In a level 2 question more is known about the topic, and there is likely to be two or more variables. Here the purpose of the research is to establish if there is a statistical relationship between the variables which have been identified. At this level, according to Brink and Wood (1994), although the researcher might have a shrewd idea of what to expect, there is not enough firm evidence to confidently predict an outcome, that would be an attribute of a level 3 question.

In a level 3 question there will be quite a lot known about the nature of the relationship between the variables in the study, enough to make a confident prediction. The purpose is to examine why a relationship exists, or to test a theory. This is achieved by manipulating the dependent variable to measure its effect on the dependent variable in an experimental design study such as a randomized control trial.

How does the researcher know how to phrase the terms of reference, and which level of question to develop? It is not an easy process, and requires practice and experience. Lo-Biondo Wood and Haber (1994) are at pains to point out that the researcher will spend a great deal of time refining the original idea into a testable research question. Although the researcher may start with a clear statement of the research problem, it is important they examine the literature carefully to establish what is known about the topic. In particular, they should seek the existence of possible relationships between the variables in the study. At this stage the researcher should examine the way similar studies have framed their questions, and the way in which they have provided concept and operational definitions for their variables as these may be useful in developing a new study.

Lo-Biondo Wood and Haber (1994) suggest the researcher should check that the terms of reference possesses the following characteristics:

- It clearly and unambiguously identifies the variables under consideration
- It clearly expresses the variables' relationship to each other
- It specifies the nature of the population being studied
- It implies the possibility of empirical testing.

The final two points are worth commenting upon. The terms of reference should give some clue as to who or what the findings will be applied to, and as a consequence, from whom or what the data will be collected. The final point suggests that it should be feasible to collect data to answer the terms of reference, that is that it is possible to collect the data in the real world.

One problem at this stage is to attempt too much in a single study without taking experience and resources into account. This danger has been described by Miles (1994) in a very readable account of her own problem in defining the research question. In considering her initial attempts at defining the terms of reference she says, 'I had made the mistake that many inexperienced researchers make and that was to try and do too much'. She concludes by reflecting back on the whole process of developing the research question and says,

> 'The main lesson that I learned from this experience of formulating a research question was that there is not a particular procedure to follow but that quite often it is a journey of discovery and indeed a problem solving exercise in itself.'

Brink and Wood (1993) also emphasize that the researcher should check very carefully that the correct level of question is developed by ruling out the existence of greater knowledge which would suggest a higher level question statement.

The hypothesis

In level 2 and 3 questions, it is usual to find a hypothesis. This can be defined as the prediction the researcher makes at the beginning of the study which links an independent variable to a dependent variable. As level 1 questions have only one variable we can see why they do not require a hypothesis.

The purpose of the hypothesis is to provide a means of demonstrating whether the researcher's prediction can be accepted or rejected. From the researcher's point of view, a hypothesis gives the study direction, as the design must take into account how the variables will be measured and the statistical way the results will be tested to see if a relationship between the variables can be established.

The hypothesis can take a number of forms, as illustrated below.

Directional/simple

Here a prediction is made as to the likely outcome between two variables, e.g. women who deliver in a midwifery led unit will have a lower level of intervention during the delivery than those on consultant led units. Here the dependent variable is the level of intervention, and the independent variable is the form of care. The hypothesis is directional because we have predicted the results will be more than, or less than that found in a comparable situation. A study with this kind of hypothesis could be a level 2 question where we are comparing midwifery led care and consultant led care, or it could be experimental where we randomly allocate women to either a midwifery led unit or consultant led unit. In this case it would be a level 3 question, as we would be deliberately manipulating the independent variable, the form of care.

Non-directional

In this kind of hypothesis, although a prediction is being made, it is not stated in which direction the outcome will be more favourable, e.g. there will be a difference in the level of intervention in those women who deliver in a midwifery led unit in comparison with those who deliver in a consultant led unit. In this example it could be that those delivered in the midwifery led unit will have less intervention, or vice versa. All that is predicted is that there will be a difference. This form is called a two-tailed hypothesis as the result could go in either of two directions (or tails). A non-directional hypothesis would be used where the researcher feels there is an association, or relationship but is uncertain of the exact nature and so keeps the direction of the findings open.

Null-hypothesis

A null-hypothesis is used in the experimental situation and is used to follow the convention in experiments that to be unbiased the researcher states that they are starting from a neutral viewpoint where they do not expect to find a difference, e.g. there will be no difference in the level of intervention at delivery between those women who deliver in a midwifery led unit or those who delivery in a consultant led unit. This is also related to statistical convention where if a difference is found, then the null-hypothesis (that there is no difference) has to be rejected. In other words, it has been demonstrated that there is a difference between the groups included in the study.

This is not an easy convention to understand. DePoy and Gitlin (1994) explain it by saying that in science it is theoretically impossible to 'prove' a relationship between two or more variables, it is only possible to reject the null hypothesis that there is no difference between two outcomes. This means there is evidence that they are different.

Complex hypotheses

This form is very similar to the simple hypothesis except there is more than one dependent variable, e.g. women who deliver in a midwifery led unit will have a lower level of intervention during the delivery and a lower level of analgesia than those who deliver in a consultant led unit. It is more usual to see hypotheses expressed separately as two simple hypotheses, as this makes them easy to test and understand.

Conducting research

For those undertaking research, the development of the research question is one of the most important steps in the research process. The preliminary stages involve ensuring that a problem area does need to be tackled through research. This concerns the relevance of the topic. It is also important to check that the study is feasible in terms of access to the sample; the resources required to carry out the study, the ethical considerations, co-operation from key people involved, and the skills of the researcher, as well as the availability of sufficient time to complete the research.

A thorough review of the literature is crucial, as this will provide valuable background information on the topic, including the possible relationships between variables that might have already been discovered. The way other authors have developed concept and operational definitions for the variables is also useful. The literature will help to identify the correct level of the question, in terms of whether it is a level 1, 2 or 3 question. The methods used in previous studies, including the way the data has been analysed, will inform the design for those intending to carry out a study.

The statement of the research question should be clear, and possible to answer through data collection. It should make reference to the sample from whom the data will be gathered, and where there is more than one variable, the nature of any relationships should be made clear.

If the level of the question is level 2 or 3, then a hypothesis may be constructed to demonstrate the prediction that is being made, and whether an association is being considered or a cause and effect relationship.

Once the research question has been constructed, along with the hypothesis if appropriate, it is worth asking, 'will the information I am collecting allow me to answer the terms of reference?'

The final check is to ensure that the research question is not too large to be undertaken in its entirety. Would it be better to take an aspect of this problem area and leave the larger questions either to a future project or to someone else?

Critiquing research

The research question, in the form of the terms of reference, is a key element in critiquing a research article. This is because so many decisions follow as a consequence of the nature of the question. The level of the question, for instance, dictates whether the design should be descriptive or experimental.

The location of the terms of reference is usually in the abstract under the title in those journals that provide an abstract. It is also commonly found just above the subheading 'method' following the review of the literature. Look for the phrase 'the aim of the research was to...' – the words stating with 'to' will form the terms of reference.

If the question is level 2 or 3, there should be a stated hypothesis, although many researchers appear to omit this. Where a hypothesis is stated, consider whether it is directional, non directional, or a null-hypothesis. Does it indicate a relationship between an independent and dependent variable in a named sample, and is the nature of that relationship stated? Is the researcher looking for an association, or a cause and effect relationship between the variables? If it is the latter, then the study should be experimental and the researcher should have manipulated the independent variable.

Whether we are dealing with a single or several variables, the researcher should provide concept and operational definitions for each one identified in the terms of reference or hypotheses. Are these clear and unambiguous?

Finally, at the end of the research article consider whether the researcher has clearly answered the terms of reference? Is there a clear conclusion that relates to the way the terms of reference was worded? Where the researcher stated one or more hypothesise, is there a clear statement as to whether these have been accepted or rejected? Most importantly, given the results of the research, do you feel the terms of reference has been adequately answered?

KEY POINTS

- Research studies revolve around collecting information to answer the terms of reference.

- The way these are constructed will influence the level of the question and the way the study is constructed.

- Research questions must be capable of being answered, they must be feasible and above all relevant.

- Level 2 and 3 questions may have a stated hypothesis which provides an indication of the prediction the researcher is making between the variables in the study.

- Hypotheses come in different forms, they can be simple, complex, directional, non-directional, or a null-hypothesis. Each one has a different purpose and should be used in the right context.

CHAPTER SEVEN

Ethics and Research

Midwives work under the midwifery rules (UKCC, 1992), and it is right that when it comes to research the midwife is accountable under the same ethical rules as other disciplines. But what are ethics and how do they relate to midwifery research? Research is not simply a process concerned with collecting information. In this chapter the ethical issues raised by research will be examined. These relate to the protection of basic human rights, and the obligations and responsibilities of the researcher in carrying out research. The main issues covered include informed consent, confidentiality, justice, and an assessment of possible benefits from the research contrasted with the possible disadvantages for the individual.

The meaning of ethics

Ethics can be defined as a code of behaviour considered correct. Talbot (1995) suggests they are 'principles of conduct governing research which are reflected by the researcher's value of, and concern for, the participants in a study'. In this way, ethics relate to two groups of people; those carrying out research, who should be aware of their obligations and responsibilities, and the 'researched upon', who have basic human rights that should be protected.

Like ethics generally, those relating to research provide a basis for deciding whether certain behaviour can be regarded as acceptable. There are a number of problems implicit in this principle, as different people may have conflicting views on what is acceptable. To overcome this dilemma, Local Research Ethics Committees (LRECs) have been set up, whose role it is to consider research projects at a planning stage to ensure that they conform to national ethical guidelines (DoH, 1991).

As medical research has been carried out far longer than midwifery research, it is not surprising that ethical principles have been developed with medical research very much in mind. This means that ethics committees often use the experimental approach, which has become synonymous with the 'scientific' approach to research, as the 'gold standard' against which others are measured.

Is it important for all midwives to know about research ethics? The simple answer is 'yes'. First, they are important in attempting to make practice research based, as they allow a judgement to be made on whether a study conforms to ethical principles. If it does not, we should suspect the researcher's honesty in all aspects of the study.

Knowledge of research ethics may also be crucial if the midwife has to act as advocate for an individual. This may include situations where an individual is involved in research that is not ethical, or where access is requested to midwifery clients for research that does not appear to be ethical (Behi and Nolan, 1995). The RCN (1993) guidelines on research, which have been adopted by midwifery, also point out that in the normal course of their work nurses and midwives may be called upon to act as witnesses to ensure that free and informed consent has been given by patients/clients prior to their involvement in research. Under these circumstances the midwife should satisfy herself that the person concerned has been given all the relevant information to make an informed decision and is not under any duress or coercion to participate.

The RCN (1993) have also pointed out that where midwives carry out research, it is more likely to be designed, completed and used in an ethically sound way if midwives understand and have thought through the implications of ethical principles.

Historical development

The content of our present ethical guidelines has been influenced by a number of internationally accepted codes on the conduct of research. These were developed following the revelation of a number of experiments that were clearly unethical and it was agreed that society should be protected from anyone who might carry out research that leads to the death or injury of those taking part. Through a series of refinements the codes outlined in Box 7.1 have influenced present day research practice in medical, nursing and midwifery research.

Nursing and midwifery guidelines

Ethical guidelines for nursing research were developed much later than medical ones. The American Nurses' Association (ANA) developed the first principles in 1968, followed by updates in 1975 and 1985. These covered not only the basic principles regarding the use of human subjects, but also examined the role of the nurse as researcher and practitioner. In Britain, guidelines were produced by the RCN in 1977 and revised in 1993. No separate guidelines exist for midwifery, although some brief advice is given in a short booklet on writing a research proposal issued by the RCM (1989). It is expected that midwives will apply the nursing guidelines to midwifery research.

The Nuremberg code

This was developed in 1947 as a result of the human experimentation carried out by the Nazi regime during World War II. The code consists of ten principles that have been influential in the conduct of research, particularly experimental research, throughout the world. The major principle relates to the necessity of obtaining informed consent from those involved in research. Although the code relates to physical interventions, it also takes account of psychological and emotional harm. One criticism of the code is that it depended on self-regulation by the experimenter.

The declaration of Helsinki

These guidelines for clinical research were developed by the World Medical Assembly at its meeting in Finland in 1964. In addition to re-emphasizing the principles of the Nuremberg Code, it developed clauses to protect subjects' human rights. An important distinction made in the declaration was between therapeutic and nontherapeutic research. Therapeutic research relates to situations where the individual may potentially benefit physically from the research, whereas in non-therapeutic research subjects probably will not benefit physically, although others may benefit in the future.

The Belmont report

The Belmont Report of 1978 highlighted what has become the three basic ethical principles of research, i) *respect for persons*, ii) *beneficence*, and iii) *justice*. One of the aims of this report was to develop guidelines on the selection of those included in the research. The report emphasizes the importance of the written consent of subjects, and the obligation of the researcher to assess the possible risk and benefits related to those who take part in the research.

Box 7.1: Major international ethical codes

Local Research Ethics Committees (LRECs)

In Britain, an important development has been the establishment of Local Research Ethics Committees (LREC) (DoH, 1991). This was an attempt to standardize the availability and functioning of ethics committees in both the public and private health sector. The role of an LREC is to consider the ethics of proposed research which involves human subjects, including those using questionnaires as a means of data collection. Most LRECs apply these guidelines to studies involving both staff and patients.

The recommended membership of these committees is eight to twelve people, composed of medical and nursing staff, general practitioners and at least two lay people. Both sexes and a wide age range should be represented, and members should have sufficient scientific and clinical expertise to make informed decisions. The guidelines made provision for the co-option of specialist advisors where necessary. The recommended term of office for committee members is three to five years (DoH, 1991).

Midwives may be approached to sit on such a committee and currently a number do have a midwife as a member. The DoH document clearly states that those sitting on such committees are not representatives of specialities or departments, but sit as individuals in their own right. This provides even more justification for midwives to understand the principles of research ethics, so that if called upon they can play a full part on such committees.

What kind of research does the LREC consider? According to the DoH (1991), an LREC must be consulted about any research proposal involving:

- NHS patients, (i.e. subjects recruited by virtue of their past or present treatment by the NHS), including those treated under contracts with private sector providers

- Access to the records of past or present NHS patients

- The use of, or potential access to, NHS premises or facilities.

The role of the LREC also covers the use of fetal material and IVF, and the recently deceased in NHS premises. The kind of projects currently not required to be considered by LRECs, even though they may have a number of the features of a research project, are those which can be considered as quality assessment studies, clinical audit or service evaluation. According to Tierney (1995), in many cases the data collection procedures and the kind of involvement by patients in these projects may be indistinguishable from those of research. She argues that it is difficult to defend the need for independent ethical scrutiny for projects called research, but exclude audit and service evaluation type studies. This, however, is likely to be an anomaly for some time to come.

In America the equivalent of the LREC is the Institutional Review Board (IRB). This is required to have at least five members of various backgrounds, who reflect professional, gender, racial and cultural diversity. Membership must include one member whose concerns are non-scientific, such as a lawyer, member of the clergy and at least one member from outside the health organization. The role of the IRB, as with the LREC, is to protect those involved in research from undue risk and loss of personal rights and dignity (LoBiondo Wood and Haber, 1994).

Basic ethical principles

Basic human rights

In this section the three basic human rights of respect for individual autonomy, protection from harm, and justice will be examined in terms of the implications they have for the researcher. In order to clarify the issues involved, these principles are presented in Box 7.2. This box outlines for each of the principles how the researcher demonstrates it has been achieved, and, just as importantly, some of the elements which would suggest that the basic human rights have been denied.

RESPECT FOR PERSON

This concept is based on the principle that an individual has the right to live their life as they choose without the control of others (Burns and Grove, 1995). It is not for us to assume that we have the right to expect an individual to take part in our research, or even that they should answer our questions (Burnard and Morrison, 1994). Individuals must be treated and respected as autonomous, that is, they should be allowed to act independently of others if their dignity is to protected.

How is this achieved? Box 7.2 illustrates that this principle is demonstrated through the researcher gaining *informed consent* from those who take part in a study. This is not a simple matter of gaining approval, or simply agreeing to take part. The important word is 'informed' consent. For this to be achieved the following should be included:

- full disclosure of details about the study;
- a statement that there is no obligation to take part, and that there are no consequences if the decision is 'no';
- assurance the individual can withdraw at any time without any negative consequences;
- confirmation of confidentiality and anonymity;
- care that all the information is understood;
- provision of an opportunity is to ask questions;
- absence of pressure, unfair inducements or coercion to take part.

Basic human principle involved	Achieved through	Denied by
Respect for person as autonomous individual	Informed consent	Right to refuse to participate or to withdraw at any point not explained. Lack of clear written information on the study given to subjects. Comprehension of information not checked. Confidentiality and anonymity not assured. Coerced to participate. Excessive or unrealistic rewards promised. Deception regarding study details. Existing relationship between researchers and subjects exploited. Covert data collection.
Protection of participants (Beneficence/non-malificence)	Risk/benefit ratio	Risks outweigh benefits. Unacceptable level of pain, discomfort or distress. Confidentiality and anonymity not protected. Access to original data not safeguarded No debriefing provided or referral to appropriate agencies offered where appropriate.
Justice	Fair selection of sample	Only vulnerable or disadvantaged group included. Captive group used, or coerced, with no opportunity to refuse or withdraw without application of sanctions.

Box 7.2: Issues involved in achieving an ethical study

What should the researcher tell a prospective subject in a study before we can say that a decision to participate was informed? A good way of thinking about this is to imagine that someone approaches you and asks if you would take part in their research. What information would you want to know before you said 'yes'?

Your answer may be quite a long list including who the people were, what organization they represented, what it will involve, particularly if there is anything invasive, painful, risky or embarrassing, the aim of the project, and what will happen to the information gathered. Anyone participating in research has the right to expect all of these queries to be answered if autonomy is to be protected. The researcher must ensure that all the details included in Box 7.3 are covered before they can claim that informed consent has been sought.

- The purpose of the study
- The identification of the researcher and their organization
- The nature of the participation (what will happen over what period of time)
- Possible risks or implications of participating, and any anticipated benefits
- Assurance of confidentiality
- Informed they need not volunteer
- Assured they have the right to withdraw at any time
- Offered the opportunity to ask questions.

Box 7.3: Information to be provided to individuals in order to achieve informed consent

An excellent example of the content of informed consent is provided by Oakley (1992) who, in the appendix to her book, includes the guidelines given to the researchers in the social support project for recruiting women into the study. This clearly satisfies the criteria set by Polit and Hungler (1997) of full disclosure without which respect for human dignity cannot be achieved.

It is not simply a matter of giving information. The researcher must ensure that the information is given in words that the individual can understand. An attempt must be made to ensure that this has been understood. This relates to the principle of *comprehension*. In some instances a judgement may have to be made on the competency of the individual to understand the information and the implications of it.

This may also apply to the circumstances under which consent is gained. For example, a woman in imminent delivery who has been taking pain relief may not really be in a position to give truly informed consent, and the implications of what she is being asked to take part in may not be fully realized at the time. An example of this is given from personal experience by Dimond (1994) who was asked for a sample of blood by an obstetric registrar shortly after her admission in labour. The registrar then returned some time later and asked that she take some gas mixture he brought. Although she at first refused, he was persistent and returned to encourage her to take the mixture on several further occasions. Her capability to make a stand against this form of intervention was reduced by the situation, and she did end up having something to which she did not truly consent. She also had numerous additional blood samples taken, and gave birth to a very drowsy baby which was almost comatose. Dimond points out the numerous elements of informed consent that were denied to her by this Registrar and highlights that part of the problem was her vulnerable state when she was persistently asked to participate.

In this respect the issue of *exploitation* must also be considered. This relates to the unfair use of an existing relationship to influence consent to take part in the study. A midwife who has had a long and intimate relationship with a woman may be exploiting that relationship by approaching her to take part in a study. It is very important, therefore, to be able to demonstrate that the consent has been made on a *voluntary basis* and is *free from coercion*, or pressure, particularly when people are *vulnerable to such approaches*.

Consideration has also to be given to gaining written consent. The DoH (1991), for instance, suggest that written consent should be required for all research except where the most trivial of procedures is concerned. However, they fail to specify what would count as a most trivial procedure. Behi (1995) also suggests that gaining written consent is an indicator of a well-designed study, while the legal advantage of gaining informed consent is emphasized by Dimond (1994).

Confidentiality and anonymity

A vital component of informed consent is the assurance of confidentiality and anonymity. Mander (1995) points out that although these two concepts are often treated as though they are synonymous, they are very different. Confidentiality is a basic ethical principle used in many professional settings, such as the law and the church. Anonymity on the other hand, Mander points out, is just one of the ways in which confidentiality is maintained. Anonymity means that steps are taken to protect the identity of an individual by neither giving their name when presenting research results, nor including identifying details which might reveal their identity. This might include such things as personal characteristics or the name of work areas where it may be possible to deduce, with reasonable accuracy, the identity of the individual.

Mander (1995) suggests that confidentiality relates to the situation or framework in which information is provided by one person to another, and that the framework should be one of trust where anonymity is assured. Confidentiality does not mean that the information will not be shared with others, as research findings frequently include comments from respondents, the key is that the person cannot be identified, and so remains anonymous.

An important aspect of confidentiality is the application of the Data Protection Act, where if names of individuals are kept on computer, the researcher must conform to the regulations of the Act. This involves the right of the individual to see the information that is kept on them, and their right not to have that information passed on to another party.

Avoiding harm

The second ethical principle is that of avoiding harm. This is discussed in the literature under a number of different headings and can be referred to as the protection of subjects, or beneficence and nonmalificence. As with professional codes of conduct, the researcher has an obligation to protect the rights and welfare of those involved in research. This means that individuals should not experience any harm as a result of the research. The Royal College of Nursing (1993) point out that in research that involves human subjects, there must be safeguards for protection against physical, mental, emotional and social harm. If there is a possibility of this, then subjects should be forewarned in order to take this into account when considering consent regarding their involvement. Protection against harm is the meaning of the words beneficence and nonmalificence. Behi and Nolan (1995) define beneficence as doing good, helping, improving and benefiting the individual, while nonmaleficence is avoiding harm to individuals.

Although midwifery researchers are unlikely to set out to inflict harm, it should be acknowledged that some form of harm may be a consequence of participating in a study. Polit and Hungler (1997) suggest that all research involves some risks, but in most cases the risk is minimal. This would apply to situations where the anticipated risks are no greater than those commonly encountered in our daily life, or those routinely experienced during physical or psychological tests or procedures. This suggests that we need to assess the type, severity and likelihood of the risks involved in a study. This is what is implied by the term '*risk/benefit analysis*', which is the way in which the protection of individuals is demonstrated at the design stage.

The type of risks that may be encountered in research are physical, psychological or emotional, although Burns and Grove (1995) warn they can also be social and financial. Where midwifery research is concerned with examining the effects of a clinical procedure, such as suturing, care of the perineum, or even something as non invasive as where the midwife places her hands during the second stage of labour, an assessment must be made of potential discomfort, pain and inconvenience. This must be weighed against the possible benefits involved, in the form of quicker healing, a return to normal functioning or quality of life as a result of the change in procedures.

The difficulty is that at the planning stage it may not be possible to say whether the change in procedure will lead to pain or discomfort, or whether there will be clear benefits as a result of the changes. It is possible, as Firby (1995) has pointed out, that individuals may be exposed to harmful effects or side effects, but the counter problem is that in a situation such as a randomized control trial, certain members of the sample may be denied accesses to beneficial effects of a new treatment or technique. In this situation the researcher must attempt to calculate the element of risks and benefits in the situation. At any time during the study, if those involved are clearly suffering, or if there is reason to suspect that continuation would result in injury, disability, undue distress, or in extreme circumstances injury or death, then the researcher has an ethical duty to terminate the study (Polit and Hungler, 1997).

It should be clear from the last statement that the protection of the individual from harm applies equally to psychological or emotional distress as well as physical consequences. This can occur not only during research involving clinical intervention, but also in surveys involving questionnaires or interviews. This may also be applied to qualitative research involving interviews or observation. These may entail an element of intrusion, embarrassment, or in some cases, such as describing a negative birth experience or the loss of a baby, a high degree of emotional distress and pain, as well as anxiety and guilt. Under these circumstances the researcher must weigh up the costs to the individual very carefully.

It does not mean that such studies should not be undertaken, as they may benefit others through a greater understanding of the experiences described. However, it does emphasize the need for the researcher to be sensitive. This may include identifying whether, in an individual's own interests, it may be wiser to terminate an interview for example. It also means that individuals should be told beforehand that there may be a possibility of painful memories being confronted in the study. If there is a likelihood of emotional distress, then the researcher must be in a position to counsel the individual, or arrange with counselling agencies to accept referrals should the need arise. It is these kinds of details that LRECs would expect to see detailed in the outline of intended research projects.

Due to the difficulties encountered with ethics committees, nursing and midwifery projects, especially those undertaken by students, have targeted staff as the subjects of their research (Miles, 1994). Although it was true that in the past many ethics committees felt that the participation of staff was a matter for the individuals concerned, LRECs now take a wider view, and staff are protected in the same way as patients.

Robinson (1996) voices her disquiet over the involvement of staff in survey research, when she talks of her concern 'at possible damage to self-esteem, work relationships or careers which could follow in the wake of the blunderbuss (or even skilled) researcher'. She points out that research on staff by a senior colleague could also compromise their ability to refuse to participate. She suggests it would be a brave person who refused to take part in a senior colleague's study, especially when everyone else on the unit had agreed.

In designing a study, the possible degrees of risk need to be considered. Where this is assessed to be no different from everyday experiences, and of a temporary duration, it would be regarded as being at a minimal level. Burns and Grove (1995) suggest that studies that include questionnaires or interviews usually involve minimal risk or can be seen as a mere inconvenience for the subjects. They go on to suggest that other studies may involve unusual levels of temporary discomfort, where subjects experience discomfort both during the study and after it has been completed. For example, an individual may be left feeling physically sore or in pain for some time later. Some qualitative studies may also have similar consequences where individuals are asked questions that involve reliving traumatic experiences or events. Extremely invasive and unreasonably painful questioning has been referred to by Robinson (1996) as 'mind rape'. Although we may feel that this is unlikely to happen within midwifery research, it is essential that we are sensitive to the possibility of respondents experiencing research in these terms.

Suggestions for avoiding psychological harm in interviews have been made by Polit and Hungler (1997). Their recommendations include the careful phrasing of questions, and the provision of debriefing sessions after an interview to permit participants to ask questions. They also suggest that the researcher should provide subjects with written information on how they may contact the researcher later, should that prove necessary or helpful.

Finally in terms of the extent of harm, it is possible that some studies could be assessed as having no anticipated elements or harm of benefits for the individual (Burns and Grove, 1995). An example would be the collection of information from records or other documents where the researcher is not in direct contact with individuals and where there is no breaking of confidentiality. Audit would fit this category as well as other studies involving records.

Justice

Justice, the third and final human principle, is rarely considered. This relates to the fair treatment of those in the study. LoBiondo-Wood and Haber (1994) suggest that an injustice occurs when benefits to which a person is entitled are denied without good reason, or when the burden of being involved in research is imposed unduly. Talbot (1995) clarifies the meaning of imposing a burden unduly by suggesting that samples and populations for a research study should be selected equally from all sections of the population. For example, groups such as those visiting antenatal clinic or those of lower social class, or midwifery staff or students should not be used merely because they are easy to locate or because they would find it difficult to refuse.

In selecting the study population, the researcher should be careful to avoid leaving themselves open to the criticism that only those people who are vulnerable to coercion or suggestion have been included. Providing they do not form a bias, all groups should stand an equal chance of being included in research projects, and should not be excluded because it is considered that have a special privileged status.

Problems in research

Firby (1995) has pointed out that as with any ethical dilemma, individuals hold differing moral views and what may seem moral to one person may not be to another. In this section some of the frequently encountered problem areas, or contentious issues will be presented so that the reader can be aware of the problems.

One contentious area relates to informed consent. Part of respecting the individual is to ensure that the purpose of the research is made clear so that the individual is in a position to truly give informed consent. But are there occasions where it is not possible to give complete details of the study without compromising the validity of the results? Polgar and Thomas (1995), for instance, warn that sometimes the researcher needs to be careful if the description of the design of the study influences the expectations and performances of the participants. For example, a study of student midwives' hand washing techniques may not be accurate if the students are told that hand washing is being observed. To gain more valid results, the researcher may have to say that they are observing routine procedures, and not draw attention to the importance of hand washing. Talbot (1995) calls this incomplete disclosure and gives the example of double blind studies where neither the researcher nor the patient knows who is receiving the experimental variable. Behi (1995) also includes covert studies in this difficult area where the covert nature of the study enhances reliability and validity. The issue of deception and the possibility of harm should always be taken into account in justifying the need for covert research methods.

Another problem area for the researcher is that of confidentiality. Although the RCN (1993) guidelines say that 'the nature of any promises of confidentiality must be strictly adhered to by the researcher', it is not always possible or in the interests of the individuals or others for this to be followed. There are instances where it is not possible to keep confidences. Examples would include where there is a greater obligation to inform others of information that has been given in confidence. Clearly where a respondent in an interview gives evidence of child abuse, the midwife researcher would have no other option but to indicate that the information could not be kept confidential. The first form of action would be to encourage the respondent to report the matter, or to give permission for the researcher to report it. If this was refused, the midwife researcher would have to report the information. The same would apply to interviews or observation of staff who were clearly involved in unsafe practices that put others at risk. Again the matter would have to be reported.

From this we can see that there can be conflict between the role of researcher and that of midwife. Where the safety of a woman or her baby is concerned, the first responsibility is to their welfare and the demands of research must come second.

In the past a documented problem area has been the actions and decisions of ethics committees who have not always understood or been sympathetic to research protocols from midwives. This particularly applies to those studies which do not take an experimental approach. Tierney (1995) suggests that, even with the development of LRECs, the problems are likely to continue as regulating the ethics of research is a complex and contentious area. Some of the problem stems from the power of doctors on such committees and their traditional narrow focus on experimental research. Oakley (1992) suggests that because much of the role of ethics committees is to assess biomedical research 'they may perform particularly badly for social research'. In her view, care should be taken in believing in the 'efficacy or ethical behaviour of such committees'. However, her extensive experience of such committees predates the establishment of LRECs. It should be admitted, however, that the overall composition or political weighting may not have changed to any great extent.

The concern of midwifery research is the way in which such committees may work as, to use Oakley's term, the 'censors of research', by essentially preventing certain types of research from being approved. The lack of familiarity of such committees with, for example, qualitative research approaches is aptly illustrated by Hunt (Hunt and Symonds, 1995) who wished to undertake an ethnographic study involving non participant observations and informal interviews over a considerable time period. The comments from the doctors on one of the ethics committees approached to grant permission show a complete lack of understanding of the conventions and approach of this type of research, despite a clear explanation provided by Hunt. She describes how, among the complaints made against her proposal, one doctor commented that 'details of the questionnaire to be used were not included', another requested clarification on the control group to be used, and another wanted more details of the statistical tests that would be used. All of these are inappropriate in ethnographic research and had been clearly indicated as such in the proposal.

This difficulty in understanding wider approaches to research is underlined by the standard submission form used by some LRECs. Tierney (1995) comments that it can be disconcerting to find that the questions on the form are framed in terms of the clinical intervention approach to research. She suggests 'the liberal use of the term not applicable' along with a carefully worded explanation where required. Unfortunately, this did not seem to work in Hunt's case.

Conducting research

This chapter has identified the main areas to consider when planning research which does not come under the heading of audit, or quality projects. All researchers are required to carry out research that reaches agreed standards of ethical conduct. These relate to the principles of:

- Informed consent
- Assessment of risk/benefit ratio
- Fair selection of subjects.

At the planning stage it is important to decide whether the proposal requires the approval of an LREC. If it does, contact the secretary for the appropriate form. A great deal of thought needs to go into completing this to ensure that it emphasizes the kinds of details that illustrate that not only the ethical principles are being followed, but also that the approach and methods used have credibility. This can be illustrated by reference to their use in similar published studies.

It must be clear in the research proposal that informed consent will be gained, and that the details of the study may be given in writing to those taking part in a study. This will include a clear statement that there is no requirement to take part in the study, and that participation is purely voluntary. It should also be clear that the individual can withdraw at any point without feeling that this may affect their care.

A form which will be used to gain written consent from each subject should be seriously considered, and included with the proposal to the LREC.

The importance of the study should be illustrated to demonstrate that the findings will make a contribution to care and service provision. Careful use of the available literature, and details of the local situation should be used to demonstrate the need for the study.

Where the applicant is new to research, it is advisable to name someone with experience, such as someone within midwifery education, or with previous research experience who will act as supervisor.

Details on steps to maintain confidentiality and anonymity should be included. If names of subjects are not required, do not ask for them. Information on the arrangements for secure data storage should be outlined. It is also wise to state that original forms, or taped interviews will be destroyed or erased once the final report has been accepted.

It is important to assure the committee that the researcher will not raise expectations that the study will result in the provision of an additional service for those who take part.

Before submitting a proposal to an LREC, it is worth discussing the proposal, particularly the ethical sections, very carefully with someone who can give advice on the subject. This may include someone who has had experience of submitting a proposal to that committee.

Even if an LREC is not involved, support from managers will be required.

Permission to start a study is one of the most important steps in the research process. There can be considerable delays and disappointment if this does not go smoothly. Do everything you can to ensure that the ethical and methodological sections of your research outline illustrate that a lot of care has gone into their construction, and is based on sound knowledge.

It is worth considering the words of Robinson (1996) who warns those about to embark on research that badly designed research is per se unethical and should not be done at all. At best it wastes patients' time and at worst it can do outright harm.

Critiquing research

Although a writer may mention some of the ethical issues covered in this section, there is not always space in an article to cover all the aspects covered in this chapter. Firby (1995) has noted that there are a number of conventions which dictate the way in which the details relating to ethics are presented. Only brief mention may be made of approval by an ethics committee, the gaining of informed consent, and the assurances of confidentiality or anonymity. This means that often the reader is left to assume that things have been carefully thought out, and that ethical safeguards have been applied.

It is reasonable for the reader to ask the following questions as a minimum:

- Was the study submitted to an ethics committee, or LREC? In the case of an American study, is there mention of an Institutional Review Board (IRB)?

- Is there evidence of freedom from bias in the way the researcher conducted the study? In particular, was the author(s) sponsored by any body or organization which might have had a vested interest in the outcome?

- Was informed consent gained?

- Were there any risks of discomfort or distress involved in taking part in the study not anticipated by the researcher, or not justified by the likely benefits to the individual/others in a similar situation?

- Did the researcher conduct the research in a sensitive manner in regard to the wording of questions and privacy afforded individuals?

- Were any foreseeable discomforts, side effects or potential risks outlined to subjects before they gave informed consent?

- Was a pilot study undertaken which may have identified any risks to the individual?

KEY POINTS

- Research is not simply a process of gathering data, but involves ethical considerations in conducting the study.

- Ethics relate to the protection of the human rights of those involved in research, and the obligations and responsibilities of the researcher. The main human rights the researcher must consider are respect for the individual, the protection against harm and justice.

- Informed consent relates to the extent to which an individual agrees to take part in a study on the basis of a clear understanding of the purpose of the research and the implications of agreeing to take part.

- The harm versus benefits ratio is the attempt to weigh up the possible disadvantages for an individual taking part in a study, against the possible positive effects.

- Justice relates to the fair treatment of all those who are potentially or actually involved in the research process.

- Each area has a local research ethics committee (LREC) whose job it is to assess the extent to which a researcher has addressed these issues in an intended research project.

- Projects that can be classified as audit usually are not required to be assessed by an ethics committee, but the researcher should still be mindful of the way the information is collected and the use to which it is put.

CHAPTER EIGHT

Surveys

Gathering data for research is exciting. However, its success depends to a large extent on the method used. This must be appropriate to the research question, and it should also be a reasonable choice for the sample group. In this chapter we shall examine the use of the survey. This can be defined as a way of gathering data by directly asking respondents for information either in the form of a questionnaire or interview.

In the following sections we will first of all examine some of the principles involved in the use of surveys, and then look at the advantages and disadvantages of questionnaires. The principles of questionnaire design will be illustrated at the end of the chapter, while the next chapter will examine the use of interviews.

The survey

The survey has become one of the most frequently used methods in the social sciences, particularly sociology (Sarantakos, 1994). Midwifery researchers have also found that this method of collecting data ideally suits many of the questions they wish to answer.

Why are surveys so popular? One reason is that they are very user-friendly. They are less intimidating for both the researcher and the subjects of the research in comparison to other forms of data collection. DePoy and Gitlin (1994) also suggest that a large amount of data can be collected quickly and cheaply with a single data collection instrument. This identifies the very practical reasons for their popularity.

As a nation we are very familiar with this method of data collection, as the media daily presents us with the results of one survey or another. Atkinson (1996) has also pointed out that in Britain, much of what is known about the nation's health, social condition, standard of living, work, education, social attitudes and behaviour is based on survey findings. In other words, they are commonly accepted as a legitimate foundation for decision making.

The basic principle on which surveys are based is that if you want to know what is going on, then the best way to find out is to ask people (Rees, 1995b). The results can be quantitative in the form of numbers, or qualitative in the form of words which identify broad issues.

Surveys can vary in a number of ways, one of the most important being the degree of structure they contain. Very structured surveys are useful if the researcher wants to check the kind of pattern involved with a certain type of activity, such as the number of women who intend to breastfeed, or the pattern of postnatal home visiting by midwives (Garcia, Renfrew and Merchant, 1994). This type of survey has the great advantage that the results are reasonably easy to analyse as it frequently involves counting the number who said 'yes' or 'no'. This method is now becoming increasingly used as the basis for audit, where repeated measures of routine information are collected.

However, the disadvantage of this method, as Couchman and Dawson (1995) observe, is that it can be a little too broad, general and superficial. They make the point that using this approach the researcher only receives what they are looking for, not what others want to say. The more unstructured the survey approach, the more in-depth the information. However, the researcher can be faced with information overload, and the answers may be very different from each other, making comparisons and summaries difficult.

The survey can also vary in relation to time period. It can take the form of a 'one-off' collection of data. This is sometimes referred to as a 'one-shot' or *'cross-sectional'* study. Here the intention is to consider how a range of people feel about a subject, or to identify their experiences in relation to a specific event or experience. It is possible to repeat data collection after a time with a different group of people to see if there has been a change. Differences in the number of women wanting a home delivery could be gathered at one point in time, and then repeated one or more years later to see if there has been a change. This is known as a *trend survey*, and works in the same way as audit where the same measurement is used at different time periods on different people to see if things have changed.

Longitudinal studies can follow the same group of people over time and keep going back to them to note any changes. This is sometimes called a panel study (Oppenheim, 1992). For instance, a study could follow women through pregnancy and the early months following the birth to assess the way in which health professionals, including the midwife, provide information.

There are two problem areas surrounding the use of surveys; the first relates to the representativeness of the sample on whom the results are based, and the second, relates to validity, or what is actually being measured. The issue relating to the sample is important as the researcher frequently wishes to generalize the findings to similar people in the wider population. For this reason surveys must try to avoid bias in the way the sample is chosen. The alternative methods of sampling will be covered in Chapter 12.

In designing the survey, it is usual to collect some basic 'demographic' details such as age, sex, or number of children, so that some comparison can be made with those in the wider population to see if they are similar. This then gives some indication of how far the sample is representative. The second question of ensuring validity is a difficult issue. One of the problems in surveys is that of the 'words/deeds dilemma' (Couchman and Dawson, 1995). This means that what people say is not necessarily what they do. There has to be an element of trust in what people say, as the truth can not always be tested by the researcher. People may be inclined to give socially acceptable answers in surveys, and so the accuracy can never be one hundred per cent. The only action the researcher can take is to try and reduce the amount of distortion produced by the data collection tool. The pilot study is one method by which this can be attempted.

Questionnaires

Questionnaires are probably the most familiar data collection tool in nursing and midwifery research. Most of us are likely to have received and probably completed one. In this section we will examine some of the advantages and disadvantages of this method and outline some of the important principles of questionnaire design.

A large number of research questions in midwifery have been answered through the use of a questionnaire. Why are they such a popular method of collecting research data? Box 8.1 suggests some of the answers.

- Cheap
- Quick
- Can reach a large geographically spread sample
- Can be quite detailed
- Low level of embarrassment or threat to both researcher and respondent
- Anonymity is protected
- Fixed choice questions easy to answer and to analyse
- Familiar method to respondents.

Box 8.1: Advantages of questionnaires

Although questionnaires can appear to be an ideal method of data collection, there are a number of considerations that may discourage a response, as Box 8.2 suggests. We do have to acknowledge that people have received so many questionnaires their motivation to complete and return yet another may not be high. For a number of reasons, the proportion returning a questionnaire can be low. If the response rate is below 50 per cent, then there is no certainty that the responses represent the views of those to whom a questionnaire has been sent. In other words, we may end up with a biased sample who may not be representative of the group we want to say something about. It is possible to send out reminders to increase the final response rate, although the return from this may also be disappointingly low.

- Questionnaires have now saturated the population
- Response rate may be low dependent on feelings on the topic
- Questionnaires are dependent on literacy and physical ability
- Responses will be influenced by the quality of the design
- There is no opportunity for clarification of questions or answers
- Fixed choice questions may not have an appropriate alternative for everyone.

Box 8.2: Disadvantages of questionnaires

One important assumption underlying the use of a questionnaire is that recipients can read and write in English. Although this may seem to suggest that the issue is one of literacy, it should be remembered that not only is literacy a problem for far more people than we may anticipate, but that many people have trouble with eyesight or problems with the ability to write because of physical problems.

A recurring disadvantage for the researcher is the frustration of receiving returned questionnaires that contain a number of unanswered questions, or where they are incomplete in some way. Once a questionnaire has been returned it is not possible to clarify answers or probe further. Finally, from the respondent's point of view, one of the frustrations of questionnaires is to find a range of answers to choose from where none of the alternatives apply to them. This raises questions of validity where a respondent is not truly describing their own views or experiences but merely choosing something the researcher has selected.

As a method the questionnaire has a number of advantages and disadvantages. They are certainly not an easy option to use in research, and have a number of restrictions and limitations. Their success depends on their design which will influence whether an individual will complete them or not. The research needs to remember the words of Oppenheim (1992) who said that a questionnaire is not just a list of questions or a form to be filled in. It is essentially a measurement tool, an instrument for the collection of particular kinds of data. For this reason the next section will consider some of the principles involved in questionnaire design.

Questionnaire design

The first stage in designing a questionnaire is to ensure that it is an appropriate method for collecting the data. Careful consideration should be given to the advantages and disadvantages outlined previously. The terms of reference should also provide some clue as to whether it is appropriate. If this includes reference to finding out what people say or do, or relates to areas where it seems that individuals themselves are in the best position to accurately supply the information, then questionnaires would seem a possible choice. The review of the literature should help to establish whether previous studies have used a questionnaire, and with what success. Once a firm decision has been made to use a questionnaire then the researcher moves into the design stage.

Designing a questionnaire is not simply concerned with writing possible questions. There are three interrelated parts to any questionnaire and each need to be constructed very carefully. These have been identified by Sarantakos (1994) as:

- The covering letter
- The instructions
- The main body.

The covering letter

Before respondents consider answering questions they need some explanation and encouragement to take part in the research. The covering letter plays a crucial role in encouraging the recipients to return the questionnaire. The letter should be persuasive but honest, and should contain some of the following elements suggested by Rees (1995c) (see Box 8.3).

- Who you are and the capacity in which you are writing (e.g. student, member of a clinical team, or manager)
- The aim of the study, in broad terms
- The reason why the person receiving it has been included in the study
- Motivation to return it (how they, or others, will benefit from completing it)
- Assurance on confidentiality
- Contact address/telephone number should they want further details or assurances (Rees, 1995c).

Box 8.3: Elements which should be included in a covering letter

Instructions

The questionnaire should start with a clear title that summarizes the purpose of the survey and should include a section marked 'Instructions'. This should simply and unambiguously tell the respondent the different ways they may be asked to respond to questions. As the respondent works their way through the questionnaire they should be in no doubt as to whether they should tick a box, circle a number or add a comment of their own. The pilot study should also provide the opportunity to test the clarity of the instructions as unless these are successful, valuable data may be lost.

The main body of the questionnaire

The crucial part of the questionnaire is the body of questions. Here we must ensure that there is as little possibility for misunderstanding or inaccuracy as possible. The respondent should find it interesting, and easy to complete, and the researcher should find that the replies provide an answer to the terms of reference. If this is to be achieved then thought has to be given to:

- The choice of questions
- The wording and structure of the questions
- The method of answering
- The analysis of the responses.

Each of these will now be considered.

THE CHOICE OF QUESTIONS

The choice of the questions will be influenced by the terms of reference and the thinking which lies behind it. Where the researcher believes that a number of variables such as parity, previous experience and attitudes towards childbirth influence a situation, these should be included in the questions. The review of the literature will also provide some pointers to relevant questions.

At the design stage there is frequently a temptation to include too many questions. The longer the questionnaire, the less likely it is to be returned. Every question should be relevant to the aim of the research. It is worth the researcher asking 'why am I including this question?' If a clear answer cannot be given, the question should be omitted. It is also an advantage to ask colleagues, and particularly 'experts' in the field, for their view on the choice of topic areas and questions.

THE WORDING AND STRUCTURE OF THE QUESTIONS

The wording and structure of the questions need special attention. First of all Box 8.3 outlines some of the basic principles of questionnaire design and although these seem straightforward, they are frequently ignored. One valuable piece of advice in questionnaire design is provided by Rees (1990) who suggests that the designer should put themselves in the place of the person completing it; will it make sense to them? Are there certain assumptions being made about the person's knowledge that may not be justified? In following this advice it may be possible to avoid mistakes such as asking questions that are not really answerable. An example would be 'do you think the birth of your baby would have been better in a different hospital?' Not only does this give no indication as to what might count as 'better', it is clearly difficult for someone to evaluate whether there would have been differences if the birth had taken place in a different unit.

Vague words are a further problem in the wording of questions. There is a need for clarity of thought that should lead to precision in the wording of questions. Words such as 'regularly' should be avoided as in 'since the birth of your baby are you able to go out regularly?' This does not explain the context in which 'going out' is placed. Does it mean shopping, visiting people or social activities? Nor would it be meaningful as a 'yes' or 'no' response, as 'regularly' could mean vastly different things to different people.

As can be seen from the list of principles in Box 8.3, one of the keys to questionnaire design is simplicity. It is important to use simple words, and avoid jargon or technical terms such as 'primiparae' and 'multiparae'. Questions should be simple and short and avoid asking more than one question in a single sentence such as:

Have you more than one child and were any of these born at home?

YES ☐   NO ☐

This should be divided into two parts, first of all it should ask 'have you more than one child and then as a further sub-question 'If 'yes', were any of these born at home? This would then appear as follows:

5 a) Have you more than one child?   YES ☐   NO ☐

    b) If yes, were any of these born at home?   YES ☐   NO ☐

It is also important to avoid biasing the individual's response through the use of leading questions or emotive words that suggest the appropriate answer, e.g.

Would you agree that the midwife kept you fully informed during the labour?

Would it be more convenient to you to attend antenatal classes in a health centre near you rather than in hospital?

This last question would be better asked in a more neutral way such as:

If you had a choice of where you could attend antenatal classes, would you choose

☐ those at St. Elsewhere

☐ those at my local health centre

☐ either one would be acceptable

THE METHOD OF ANSWERING

The method of answering questions can take a number of forms. The example above is called multiple choice, where the respondent chooses one of the alternatives offered. This falls into the category of closed questions as opposed to open questions. In open questions the respondent is not offered alternatives to choose from but is left to phrase the answer in their own words. An example of an open question would be the following:

What did you hope to gain from attending antenatal classes?

Open questions work very well where respondents are used to expressing themselves in writing, but we should keep in mind that this method may not be acceptable or productive for everyone.

Open and closed questions have their advantages and disadvantages. For instance, although closed questions have the advantage of simplicity, they may influence the respondent by suggesting answers that they may not have thought of without the prompt of the fixed-choice alternatives. The open question then has the advantage of the respondent using terms and options which they feel describe their own experiences or views, rather than using those offered by the researcher. The disadvantage of open questions is the large amount of data that has to be analysed and coded before any kind of summary or identification of issues takes place. The ideal compromise is to have a mix of open and closed questions, which maximize the advantages of both forms of question.

One method of increasing the sensitivity of closed questions is through the use of scaling techniques (Oppenheim, 1992). Although we often think of closed questions as having a yes or no answer, where attitude or opinion is concerned, how people feel about an issue or statement may lie anywhere along a continuum. This can be dealt with using a Likert scale, which is named after the American Rensis Likert, who first introduced them. These can take three forms and relate to:

- Agreement
- Evaluation
- Frequency.

In the case of agreement scales, statements in either a positive or negative form are given and the respondent is asked to make a choice between five alternatives ranging from strongly agree to strongly disagree. Smith (1996), in her study of women's beliefs about the role of the midwife in home and hospital deliveries, used this approach, and her results section clearly illustrates the use of statements with alternative choices. Fictional examples are shown below:

i) agreement

I feel that pain relief in labour should be taken as a last resort

☐ strongly agree   ☐ agree   ☐ undecided

☐ disagree   ☐ strongly disagree

ii) evaluation

The information I received from the midwife about the alternative forms of pain relief was

☐ excellent   ☐ very good   ☐ undecided

☐ poor   ☐ very poor

iii) frequency

I get feelings of panic when I think about looking after the baby

☐ always   ☐ sometimes   ☐ rarely

☐ never

In the last example four alternatives have been used as these seem to cover the main alternatives. The inclusion of 'never' removes the necessity to include a neutral mid-category. Some people argue that with the first and second alternatives above, the mid-category of 'neither' should be removed to prevent people choosing a neutral option and sitting on the fence. From experience, this has never been the case in practice, and it should be remembered that there should be an alternative that applies to everyone. Sometimes a mid-category could be a legitimate choice and should be respected.

The statements or 'items' in the Likert scale should be a mix of those expressed positively and those expressed negatively to prevent respondents simply putting a tick in the same column each time without really thinking about the question. So for instance, the following two examples may be used in a satisfaction questionnaire.

The midwife was too busy to answer my questions (negative item)
I felt confident with the midwife who conducted the delivery (positive item)

The order of these statements should not follow a set pattern, for instance, alternately positive and negative, providing there is an equal number of each kind of statement they should be presented in a random order.

A similar technique to the Likert scale is to use a visual analogue scale (VAS) which is a line drawn across the page, usually ten centimetres, with opposite words at each end. The respondent is asked to place a cross on the line to correspond with how they feel. This can either be calibrated with lines at centimetre points, or can be assessed during the analysis by laying over the line a clear piece of plastic which is calibrated. This approach is often used in relation to pain. An example would be:

Mark with a cross on the line how you would describe your pain now

worst pain
imaginable   no pain at all

⌐_____⌐

THE ANALYSIS OF THE RESPONSES
The analysis of both the Likert scale and the visual analogue scale can be treated in a similar way by allocating a numeric value for the chosen response. In the case of the Likert scale the score of 5 can be allocated for 'strongly agree' answers, 4 for 'agree', 3 for 'neither agree/disagree', 2 for 'disagree' and 1 for 'strongly disagree' when the statement is in the positive. When the statement is expressed in the negative, the reverse order of numbering would be applied (i.e. strongly disagree to the statement 'the midwife did not have time to answer my questions' would be scored 5 to show there was a positive response to the midwife). An overall score for all the Likert questions can then be calculated for each person. It is also possible to give an average score for everyone in the sample. So for instance, an average of 4.2 for the statement 'I felt confident with the midwife who delivered me' would suggest that there was a high degree of satisfaction as the average was between the 'agree' and 'strongly agree' point on the scale. In the same way the points on the visual analogue scale could be divided into ten sections with each section given a score from one to ten, where ten could be allocated to the positive end of the scale and one to the negative.

In questions requiring a 'yes' or 'no' answer, the responses can be expressed as a proportion of the total in terms of the percentage giving each response. The method of analysis should be carefully thought out at the design stage, and tested in the pilot and not left until the questionnaires start arriving.

Conducting research

Although a survey provides quick and easy access to a large amount of data, the researcher should be cautious in the use of the questionnaire. This is because it is not always an appropriate method for many people for whom writing is either not an easy or welcome mental activity, or for those who have a physical condition, such as a visual problem or writing problem. We have also to remember that even for those who are used to expressing themselves on paper, questionnaires have almost reached saturation point, and the motivation to complete and return a detailed questionnaire may be low.

Consideration must be given to the nature of the terms of reference, the sample under consideration, and the possible advantages of using an alternative method such as interviews. The question of ethics should also be raised at this stage, as thought needs to be given to the possible harm through upset, anxiety or guilt caused by certain kinds of topic areas. These may include the loss of a baby or the birth of a baby with a medical problem that may be thought to relate to maternal behaviour, such as smoking or dietary intake. Robinson (1996) warns that personal questions can cause distress to patients and arouse anxieties that may linger. Care should be taken, then, where the respondent may confront emotionally sensitive issues when they may be in a vulnerable mental state, and may have no one to help them through the distress caused by the questionnaire.

Where the decision to use the questionnaire is appropriate, it is important to avoid believing it is all a matter of writing appropriate questions down on paper. The three elements of covering letter, instructions and main body of the questionnaire need careful planning and design. The review of the literature will help identify appropriate topic areas, and may even give some pointers as to the kind of questions that have worked well in other studies. In selecting the wording of the questions the researcher must keep validity and reliability in mind. The two important questions which need to be constantly addressed are:

- What am I trying to measure (validity)?
- How accurately will this question measure it (reliability)?

The basic principles of questionnaire design should then be rigorously followed. Decisions on how the data resulting from each question are to be displayed in a final report should be considered at the question design stage. If you feel you may need statistical advice, it is at this stage that it should be sought.

It is important to make the questions as clear and as straightforward as possible. This means using simple language and simple sentences. Midwifery or medical jargon and abbreviations should be avoided as much as possible. It is not easy for the researcher to spot vague terms and ambiguity, so it is important to ask others to comment at the design stage.

A questionnaire should be interesting and enjoyable for your respondents to fill in. There should be variety in the way the questions are asked or require to be answered. The most frustrating experience for a respondent is to find that the choice of words clearly betrays the researcher's preconceived assumptions or personal agenda. This can be revealed through the use of emotive words such as 'better', 'disappointed', 'acceptable', and so on.

A pilot *must* be undertaken. In the pilot it is important to have a good cross-section of the kinds of people who will be included in the main study. This is perhaps just as important as the size of the sample. It is a good idea to produce a report based on the analysis of the data from the pilot to provide experience of moving from raw data to data presentation and analysis. At this point serious shortcomings in the design of some questions, especially the method of answering, can be revealed. It is worth ending with the words of Oppenheim (1992) who said that every aspect of a survey has to be tried out beforehand to make sure that it works as intended.

Critiquing research

Questionnaires are a popular method of data collection in midwifery. The danger is that we have become so familiar with them that we rarely stop and challenge their use. We do need to ensure that the researcher has given a clear rationale for the choice of questionnaire rather than the usually more effective method of interviewing. Where the sample is geographically spread, or where there is already a relationship between the researcher and the respondents that may influence the results of an interview, then questionnaires are a good choice. It is worth thinking about any ethical issues raised by the use of the questionnaires, and whether this has been addressed by the researcher. For instance, we would be unhappy where a questionnaire was used to explore feelings about a stillbirth or abortion, or similar subjects that may result in upset, anxiety or needlessly raising feelings of guilt, confusion or regret.

The space provided in some journals does not permit the inclusion of an entire questionnaire, so that we cannot always judge the quality of the design. Sometimes tables do provide a good indication of both the question wording, and the method of answering (Smith, 1996). Where possible, place yourself in the position of the respondents and ask was there any possibility of ambiguity, or misunderstanding? Are the questions in any way leading, for instance, through the use of emotive words that suggests how the researcher felt about the topic?

What evidence is there that the researcher addressed the issue of reliability of the questions, especially if they were designed for the study and had not been used previously by other researchers? Was the accuracy of the questions tested through a pilot study, for instance? In regard to validity, how do we know the questions were measuring what they were supposed to measure? Did the researcher develop some of the questions from previous research, or were experts in the field approached to comment on the appropriateness of the topics for the study?

Finally we should consider the interpretation that the researcher puts on the results. Are the results strong enough to support the statements made by the researcher? We should also be aware of the words/deeds dilemma, in that what people say they do, may not be what they do in practice. In other words we should always be somewhat cautious in treating self-report data as if it were 'the truth'.

KEY POINTS

- Questionnaires enable a large amount of data to be collected quickly and cheaply. They have the advantage of being familiar to a majority of the population, and compared to other forms of data collection are a reasonably non-threatening medium for both the researcher and respondent.

- The response rate is variable. Where it falls under 50 per cent, it is difficult to be certain that the responses received are representative of the sample to whom the questionnaire was sent.

- There is also the problem that questionnaires have been used so much in the past that people are now less likely to return them. Serious consideration should be given as to whether this is the most appropriate method. In particular, the ethical issue of harm should be considered where the questions may produce emotional upset, regret, anxiety or confusion.

- Designing a questionnaire involves three elements; the covering letter, the instructions and the body of the questionnaire. There are clear guidelines that should be followed in the construction of questions. The importance of avoiding bias and ensuring reliability and validity must be stressed.

- It should be remembered that the basic premise of questionnaire design is that the respondent can read and write, and is fluent in the English language. For one reason or another there is a proportion of the population who will always be excluded where questionnaires are used to collect research data.

- A pilot study is a good indicator of rigour in the use of questionnaires.

CHAPTER NINE

Interviews

Survey methods make a great use of interviews as a way of collecting data. As we shall see, they are similar to questionnaires in many respects including the variety of structure they use. It is worth remembering that questionnaires can suffer from the major problem of poor response rate. Certainly for the mothers of new babies, sitting down to complete a questionnaire may be difficult to achieve. Not only can questionnaires be difficult to fit into a hectic lifestyle, but they are now almost an over-used medium for collecting research data. There is so much 'junk-mail' received in the post that it is very easy to include questionnaires in this category.

Interviews have a great deal to offer midwifery research, as the type of data it produces tends to be richer, and has more depth than is generally possible with questionnaires. Interviews also make use of the midwife's professional skill of sensitively collecting information through a conversational type of medium which is more familiar to people. It can also increase the range of people included in a study.

In this chapter we shall examine some of the features of interviews, especially their advantages and disadvantages, and we shall pay particular attention to some of the skills involved in interviewing.

Definition

Interviews consist of data gathering through direct interaction between a researcher and respondent where answers to questions are gathered verbally. They can take the form of face to face encounters or the use of the telephone. Although usually conducted on a one to one basis, they can be carried out with a group of individuals. They have a certain degree of acceptability with respondents, this is because, as McKie (1996) points out, they capitalize on the most natural form of social communication, the conversation.

Structure of interviews

Interviews vary in a number of ways. One of the most obvious is the degree of structure. They can range from a highly structured format, where they virtually take the form of reading out questions from a questionnaire, and recording the answers. This approach is used in survey designs which concentrate on the production of quantitative data (Newell, 1994). Here, the list of questions is known as an *interview schedule*. The advantage of this format are emphasized by Newell (1994) who presents the following list:

- It is easier to code the responses and analyse and interpret the data
- The uniformity of the questioning enables the results to be analysed quantitatively and tested for statistical significance
- It is easier to train interviewers to use a structured interview schedule as written guidance on its use is provided
- Producing a structured interview schedule encourages the researcher to crystallise his or her thoughts and ensure that clear definitions and precise questions are developed.

The disadvantage of a highly structured approach is that there is little scope for spontaneity and depth of information. It can also be very superficial leaving us with little understanding of a situation. Newell (1994) also points out that of all interviewing techniques, the structured interview is the one which is most distinct from normal conversational interaction. She also suggests that the disadvantages include omitting areas relevant to a study because the researcher has not considered them, and forcing respondents to choose from a list of closed options, none of which really apply.

At the other end of the interview continuum is the unstructured, or non-standardized interview, where the line of questioning can be developed very much as seems appropriate within the confines of each particular interview.

The advantage of this approach is that the interviewer responds very much to the experiences or situation of the respondent, and the information is not forced or channelled into a limited number of options. In this way, as Burnard and Morrison (1994) point out, the respondent has much more control over how the interview will proceed. This has its advantages in situations where the researcher knows the broad area to be covered, such as the decision on method of infant feeding, but is unsure of the exact points to be covered. Using a qualitative method, issues can be explored in an unrestricted manner and so illuminate the topic from the respondents point of view (McKie, 1996).

The disadvantage of the approach is that this loose structure makes it very difficult to summarize a number of interviews together, as they may cover very different topics and issues. Analysis can thus be very difficult. Rather than numbers, the researcher is more likely to produce quotes from respondents (Too, 1996) or extended dialogue between the researcher and respondents (Oakley, 1992).

In between these two extremes we have semi-structured interviews, which are a mixture of the two. They contain some standard questions, which are asked of everyone, but there is also the flexibility to probe and explore areas that seem appropriate to the individual concerned. An *interview guide* is the name given to the checklist of questions, or key words used by the interviewer in this kind of situation. Burnard and Morrison (1994) point out that this approach breaks up the strict format of the structured approach and can yield 'richer' data. The advantage for the researcher is the ability to get closer to the accurate views, feelings and experiences of the respondent. The excitement of developing this picture from the respondent's point of view is brought out in the following statement from Rose (1994):

'Semi-structured interviewing, therefore, contains an element of adventure, a step into the unknown, into the life and feelings of another human being.'

This mixture of open and closed questioning appears to be an ideal compromise, enabling the production of both quantitative and qualitative data. It should be remembered, however, that these three different forms of interviews are imaginary points along a continuum. Most interviews will not be located neatly at one of these points, but somewhere between the two extremes, depending on the nature of the research question, and the way the researcher has decided to answer it.

Advantages of interviews

Why choose interviews as a data collection method? There are a number of very clear advantages to using interviews as can be seen from Box 9.1. According to Polit and Hungler (1991), interviews suffer from fewer weaknesses than questionnaires, and their advantages far outweigh those of questionnaires. They have a higher response rate, are suitable for a wider variety of individuals than questionnaires, are less likely to lead to misinterpretations of the questions, and provide richer data than questionnaires. This is because the choice of answers usually has fewer restrictions than the visual prompts provided by questionnaires, unless a strict structured interview is used. The presence of the interviewer can also be an asset as she can encourage the provision of complete and accurate answers. This has been recognized by Burns and Grove (1995) who suggest that interviews allow the researcher to explore a greater depth of meaning than can be obtained with other methods.

Interviews have a particular relevance in midwifery as they provide an opportunity to pursue a woman centred approach to issues and situations. This is particularly the case in semi-structured and unstructured interviews as 'they allow informants to tell their own stories, in the way they choose, and to express their feeling directly, without the constraints of rigid pre-determined questions' (Rose, 1994).

- Responses can be gained from a wide range of people including those who have problems with literacy, visual problems, and are suitable for mothers and health professionals, who have very little time to complete questionnaires
- Response rate is usually higher than questionnaires
- The interviewer has control over the situation and can reduce misunderstandings or missed questions
- Most of the data is usable
- In-depth responses can be gained
- Data is immediately available
- Overall better quality data in comparison to questionnaires.

Box 9.1: Advantages of interviews

As with all the other methods presented in this book, we also have to be aware of the disadvantages of interviews. The main issues are outlined in Box 9.2. A number of these relate to the practicalities of the technique. They require a great deal of time per interview in terms of both gathering the data and its analysis, particularly where the interview is semi-structured, or unstructured.

The other important difficulty is the influence of the interviewer. The fact that this is a social situation means that the characteristics of each of the individuals concerned can play a part in the reliability and validity of the information produced. There is inevitably a conscious or subconscious influence on the selection of information by the respondent where the interviewer is a midwife, no matter how much they encourage respondents to 'tell it as it is'. Hardy and Mulhall (1994) draw attention to this, and question the implication of interview situations where the interviewer is a health professional, and the respondent a member of the public. The question they pose is 'does the status of the interviewer influence the type of answer where the interviewer is seen as a powerful figure when socially desirable answers may be given?' The element of 'social desirability' means that people say what they feel would be approved by the interviewer, as the kind of answer that would gain social approval.

In a similar vein, Fielding (1994) identifies a number of problems related to the social aspect of the interview and the selection of material by the interviewee. He suggests that respondents tend to rationalize the situations or choices they describe and present an explanation based on logical reasoning rather than admitting that it may be based on emotional or illogical factors. Respondents may also be afraid of being 'shown up' and so adapt the truth somewhat. He also suggests that people can be over polite and become eager to impress, or attempt to anticipate the kind of answers they imagine the interviewer wants to hear. All these elements will tend to have a negative effect on the validity of the data collected through interviews.

- Interviewing is a highly skilled activity which requires careful training and practice
- It is time consuming and costly to carry out and analyse in comparison to questionnaires
- There is a danger of respondents providing 'socially acceptable' answers
- Respondents can be influenced by the interviewer's status, characteristics or behaviour
- Respondents can feel put on the spot, 'tested', or worry they will 'look a fool' if they answer completely honestly
- Some respondents may not be used to expressing their feelings openly to others.

Box 9.2: Disadvantages of interviews

The list in Box 9.2 illustrates the role of the interviewer's skills, and these will be considered in the next section.

The interview

> 'Interviewing is rather like marriage: everybody knows what it is, an awful lot of people do it, and yet behind each closed door is a world of secrets.'

The above comment from Oakley (1981) illustrates why we need to examine the interview in detail. Interviewing is a skill frequently practised outside the gaze of those who may be able to learn from those who do it well. Although interviewing sounds a deceptively easy activity, consisting of asking questions and receiving answers, like everything else in research, things are never that easy. You can, however, overcome some of the difficulties if you are aware of the pitfalls and follow some basic principles.

Barker (1996) suggests that interviews are one of the commonest and perhaps easiest means of data collection at our disposal. By this he means that they appear familiar and follow the turn-taking principle of ordinary conversation, or professional questioning. However, the similarity stops there. Oppenheim (1992), one of the foremost writers on interviews, makes the point that the interview is not an ordinary conversation, and suggests that probably no other skill is as important to the survey research worker as the ability to conduct good interviews, a point that can be applied to all types of interviews.

One of the first considerations in carrying out an interview is the location and characteristics of the environment in which the interview takes place. The respondent should feel relaxed and comfortable. There should be as few disturbances and distractions as possible whilst the interview takes place. Although many people provide the best information in their own home, the interviewer's control over the setting is drastically reduced. Despite interruptions having an impact on the flow of information, sometimes this may be inevitable, especially with a young baby around. Under these circumstances it is important the interviewer does not show any irritation or exasperation. Wherever the interview takes place, simple things such as ensuring that the sun is not shining in the respondent's eyes, and that they are comfortable is important, as this will affect the quality of the information produced.

The interviewer's appearance also needs consideration, if the possibility of producing socially desirable answers is to be minimized. The way the interviewer is dressed or items they are wearing could act as distractions, or indications of possible personal beliefs or values. Where possible the interviewer's appearance should be relatively nondescript.

It is also important that the interviewer states the approximate length of time the interview may take and ensures that the respondent is not worried about other responsibilities or appointments that may distract them as the interview lengthens.

The nature of the interview will also be influenced by the method of recording the answers. Here the two options are making written notes, or using a tape recorder. Both have their advantages and disadvantages. Written notes are not as intimidating as using a tape recorder, and the interviewer is not worried by background noise. There is also little risk of technology letting the researcher down, although it is important to have a good supply of pens or pencils that are in good working order! The disadvantage of writing is the inability to maintain eye contact with respondents. This can be a difficulty for both the interviewer and interviewee. It can feel somewhat like making a police statement rather than an interview. There is also an inevitable 'loss' of information, as it is rarely possible to write down everything that is said.

Tape recorders have the advantage of leaving the interviewer free to concentrate on the conversation rather than trying to speed-write everything that is said. The ability to maintain eye contact can also be very important in interviews on sensitive topics. Apart from the problem of background noise, tape recorders are successful in capturing almost all of the comments from the respondent in their own words. This can be a crucial advantage, particularly in qualitative research. The disadvantages of tape recorders include the fact that some respondents find them intimidating, and they are an additional worry for the interviewer, in case something goes wrong with them, such as the tape jamming, or the batteries running out. The resultant interviews can also take a long time to transcribe ready for analysis.

Interview skills

McKie (1996) suggests that there are a number of factors which affect the outcome of the interview as a method. These are divided into objective and subjective qualities of the interviewer. The objective qualities include the interviewer's age, gender, social class, manner of dress and accent. Subjective factors include the ability of the researcher to quickly establish rapport and maintain a smooth flow within the interview. Apart from choice of dress, there is little the interviewer can do about the objective qualities, so it is the subjective factors which need to be examined in more detail.

According to Barker (1996), the quality of the information generated from the interview is dependent, to a great extent, on the behaviour of the interviewer. What can the interviewer do to increase the chances of a productive interview? Box 9.3 outlines some of the principles the researcher should be aware of in the form of the acronym S-O-L-E-R.

S – it to the side of the interviewee facing in, at just less than ninety degrees
O – pen posture
L – ean forwards slightly to indicate active listening
E – ye contact
R – elax

Box 9.3: Principles in interviewing

A number of these items relate to the elements of non-verbal communication. These enhance the establishment and maintenance of 'rapport', which can be defined as an understanding and close relationship between both parties. The physical position of the interviewer in relation to the interviewee is important; if they are square-on, almost in a head-to-head position, the respondent may feel it is more like an interrogation rather than a relaxed conversation. Sitting slightly to the side of the individual where eye contact can be made helps to establish the right atmosphere. It is important that this is at a comfortable distance from the individual, so that they do not feel that their personal space is being restricted, or invaded.

In order for people to feel valued it is important that the person with whom they are talking maintains comfortable eye contact with them, and leans slightly forward to indicate that they are listening. The interviewer should avoid crossing their arms or legs, which may suggest that they are nervous, or keeping certain information secret from the respondent. The key element is to relax. If the interviewer is relaxed, it will encourage the respondent to similarly relax.

The role of the interviewer

An important issue within midwifery is the role that the interviewer takes in relation to the interviewee. Traditionally, research texts have warned the researcher to avoid becoming involved with the content of the respondents replies, in order to maintain objectivity and to avoid leading the respondent in any way. Polit and Hungler (1991), for instance, state that 'an interviewer is a neutral agent through whom questions and answers are passed'. Although we can agree that the interviewer should avoid influencing the respondent, we should question whether it is possible to remain completely neutral in an interview, and what the consequence of that would be for the respondent?

Oakley (1981) has drawn attention to the one-sided view of the interviewer in traditional, male research texts, and suggests that women interviewing women is a contradiction in terms. Although traditionally interviewers have been warned to keep their social distance from their subjects, Oakley (1981) suggests that the relationship should be far more equal, and that the researcher owes it to her subjects to give as much as she takes. By this she means that where an interviewee asks a question of the researcher, this should be answered as honestly and openly as possible. This then counter-balances the one way direction of information that has characterized interviews in the past.

From a feminist perspective of research it is perfectly legitimate to share personal information or to provide information when asked, rather than to see this as endangering the objectivity of the data. For instance Buckeldee (1994), in her research comments on how she handled the situation where respondents wanted to continue the social interaction with the researcher although data collection had been concluded, stated:

> '...there are difficulties of leaving a respondent after the interview is over, particularly where the respondent clearly wants to carry on talking – Particularly in the early interviews my feelings were that, having helped me with my study, it was only fair to spend time talking with participants if they wanted this.'

It is interesting that some feminist researchers have used the term 'guided conversation', rather than interview, which according to Bergum (1991) implies a discussion and best captures the attitude of two-way interaction. It is important, then, for the midwifery interviewer to feel that interviews can be two way, and that information can, and indeed, should be shared with those who are happy to give freely of their time for the benefit of the researcher.

When things go wrong

Inevitably things may go wrong during an interview, and it is just as well to be prepared for them. Common problems include an incomplete answer to a question, where the respondent only gives part of an answer. Other problems include wrongly anticipating a question and so providing an answer that is not appropriate to the question. The following suggestions from Moser and Kalton (1971) can be very useful techniques to correct the situation.

- Use of the expectant pause
- Use of the expectant glance
- Repeat part of the answer
- Repeat original question.

The first two suggestions of an expectant pause or glance suggest to the respondent that it is still 'their turn' to speak, and this will usually be taken as a cue to continue with their conversation. However, care has to be taken, with both of these techniques, as the expectant pause can turn into an embarrassing silence, and the expectant glance can turn into a nervous twitch!

Repeating part of the answer can also be a signal to continue, and is very useful when taking written notes, as it allows the respondent to receive feedback that the information has been received.

Repeating the original question can alert the interviewee that perhaps the original question was misheard, and will allow them to correct this by providing an answer that corresponds with the question posed.

We should also remember that things can go wrong in an interview because it is potentially a stressful situation for both interviewer and interviewee. Both may suffer from what Morse and Field (1996) describe as 'stage fright'. That is, they may restrict what they say or not act naturally because they are intimidated or over-awed by their involvement in research. This feeling can be increased where a tape recorder is being used. The interviewee's reaction to this situation can be quickly spotted when the interview becomes more like a quick question and answer session, rather than the establishment of a considered and in-depth answer. The replies may be very short one word or sentence answers, or the respondent might keep saying they do not remember, or it never bothered them.

Morse and Field (1996) also point out that some of the problem may lie with the interviewer. If intimidated they may hurry the interview along so the interviewee does not get sufficient time to reflect on the answer before the next question is asked. In this situation the interviewer needs practice in interviewing, so that they are comfortable with the technique. Where a tape recorder is used, it should be placed discretely out of eye-line for both of them, so they are not intimidated by its presence.

All the issues in this section underline the conclusion that interviewing is a highly skilled activity. The interviewer should be familiar with the content of the interview, and should have practised with it several times before it is piloted under natural conditions. The rewards of interviews are many, and it is worth considering the way in which research based on interviews have illuminated many of the important issues in midwifery.

Conducting research

Interviews should be considered when the research question depends on self report which can be enhanced by a face to face situation. This can be where the respondent has not considered the subject in any depth and may not feel their views as important enough to return a questionnaire. Similarly, they should be considered where the topic may be one capable of great depth and a questionnaire would be too superficial a method. They should also be considered where the researcher intends to explore the topic through the eyes of the respondents and wants respondents to recount their experiences in some depth in their own words. All this is summed up by Oppenheim (1992) who suggests that the longer, the more difficult and the more open ended the question schedule is, the more we should prefer to use interviews.

Interviews can be used as a stand alone method or used in addition to other methods of data collection such as observation (Phillips and Davies, 1995).

Once the interview has been decided as the appropriate tool, the researcher must consider the degree of structure it will contain ranging from structured, through to semi-structured and unstructured. Whichever degree of structure, the researcher must ensure they are fully trained and experienced in undertaking the role of interviewer. This is essential, according to Buckeldee (1994), if interviews are to become a truly fruitful form of data collection. She suggests practising the interview with peers or other researchers, or listening critically to tapes of one's own interviews.

In the interview setting, it is important to be aware of the impact of interruptions and distractions. The body language of the interviewer is crucial in helping the respondent to relax in what can be a very stressful and intimidating situation. Although there are many skills involved in the interview, it is worth remembering the advice of Morse and Field (1996) who say that good interviewers listen. This is important where there are interruptions or where the interviewee makes a decision to go down a particular road in the interview. Where it is clear that the respondent has decided to follow one line of a description, or account, rather than another, it is important for the interviewer to consider whether they need to bring them back to that point and explore the other alternative. Where an interruption occurs the interviewer may have to help the respondent to return to the place that had been reached. This is why Morse and Field (1996) say a good interviewer is someone who can keep track of the story.

The complexity of the interview situation has been emphasized in a characteristically vivid way by Oppenheim (1992) who suggests that the interviewer has to engage in 'a spot of rapid mental traffic management' during the interview, as it is not possible to follow every option the interviewee offers. The options have to be stored, sorted and returned to if important. Rose (1994) also emphasizes this point by saying that each interview occurs only once, so the interviewer must have the ability to home in on the chance remark where further probing may produce a wealth of extra data.

Anything can happen in a free flowing interview. An important warning from Morse and Field (1996) is that while telling their 'story', respondents will relive their experiences, including the emotional responses. If a memory is stressful or painful, the respondent may experience anger, fear, sadness or upset. Under these circumstances the interview may have to be abandoned or delayed until the respondent makes a decision as to whether they want to continue, or the interviewer feels that it would be in the respondents best interest to abandon or reschedule the session. However, some people find these emotional moments therapeutic. Respondents can sometimes feel grateful for the opportunity for someone at last to listen to their experiences and feelings.

Where an interview is particularly intense it is possible for the feelings of closeness to lead to the interviewee revealing what Morse and Field (1996) refer to as 'secret information'. It should be remembered that where the interviewer is a midwife, the professional code of conduct does not allow all information to be kept secret. Examples would be anything related to child or mother abuse or neglect, or a report of poor professional conduct. Under these circumstances the midwife cannot adopt a researcher role of keeping the information confidential but has a duty to report it. Under these circumstances, where a respondent indicates that they want to share something which they indicate is particularly confidential, the midwife interviewer must stop them and make their own position clear before the respondent says something which they may later regret.

These points emphasize the exhausting nature of interviews, especially those touching on very sensitive areas. Buckeldee (1994) talks honestly about this aspect of her own work in nursing where she says 'undertaking such interviews can be tiring and completing each interview frequently left me exhausted'. For this reason Rose (1994) wisely suggests that research cannot be undertaken in a vacuum, and it is important for the researcher to talk about the problems and experiences, either with an academic supervisor, or a close colleague.

Finally, at the end of the interview Morse and Field (1996) suggest that the interview should end with the questions 'Is there anything you would like to ask me?' and 'Is there anything else I should have asked you?'

Critiquing research

In critiquing a research article that has used interviews, the first question to ask is, 'was it an appropriate choice of data collection?' In other words, would the disadvantages of the interview setting have suggested that an alternative method may have been more appropriate? One problem with many research reports is that it is difficult to get an idea of the conditions under which the interview took place, so we have no idea of the possible strength and weakness that may have influenced the reliability of the interview. An excellent exception is the work of Bluff and Holloway (1994) where a great deal of detail is provided on the environment in which the interviews took place, and the details of the interviews themselves.

In most instances, although the person undertaking the interview may be named, we have little idea how they were dressed. The problem we should be alert to is whether the interviewer was a midwife and known to the respondents, and whether they were in uniform. Both these factors may influence the results.

We also need some indication of the degree of structure in the interview which may have encouraged or curtailed the views of the respondent, and the language in which they could respond; the more the interview was structured, the less views could be expressed in the respondent own words.

The presentation of results is also important. Although some selection and editing is inevitable, the more that has taken place, the less authentic the results. A good positive example of this is the work of McIntosh (1988) who tries to present the results of his interviews with Glaswegian women as accurately as possible using their exact words and their speech patterns. The following is an example of how one woman spoke about the forthcoming birth of her baby:

> 'I'm just terribly excited. It's like gettin' a Christmas present. I'm no' worried about anything. Ah just think it'll be great.'

The richness of the data is apparent from this quote which would lose a great deal of its impact if it had been 'corrected' and presented in 'plain English'. In some examples the person providing the quote is indicated by either a number in brackets, e.g. (6) or by a pseudonym as in the case of Too (1996). It is worth checking that the quotes are taken from a cross-section of respondents, and not the same articulate but perhaps unrepresentative few who are being used to illustrate the points.

An important note on which to end is the reminder that interviews and questionnaires, only relate to what people say, and not necessarily to what they do. This is emphasized by Fielding (1994), who states that the major assumption made in interview research is that what people say is an indicator of thought and action, and that attitudes are assumed to be a direct influence on behaviour. However, the relationship between words and action is problematic. We would need further evidence, in the form of observational data, to convince us that people do what they say they do, or that their stated attitudes influence their choices and behaviour.

We should also acknowledge that people's memories of past events can be selective, and in some instances, inaccurate (Fielding, 1994). In looking at assessments of midwifery services it is also important to remember that on the whole patients will express a preference for what they receive and know (Robinson, 1996). This explains why, when comparing a potentially more beneficial form of a service against a group receiving a traditional form of service, the levels of satisfaction can appear very similar. This is because the 'traditional' group can rate their care highly because of its familiarity, and not necessarily its inherent quality.

KEY POINTS

- Interviews have many advantages over questionnaires as a means of data collection. In midwifery they also have the advantage that they are compatible with a woman centred approach to care. They can be used to collect quantitative data using a structured interview schedule, or qualitative data using a semi-structured, or unstructured format.

- Semi-structured, and unstructured interviews have the advantage that they can collect a rich quantity of data through the prolonged and interactive format of the interview. They provide a unique view of events as seen by those receiving services, or those experiencing parenthood. The results are frequently unexpected and illuminating, and can differ from the perspective of health professionals.

- There are a number of disadvantages to interviews. They are costly and time consuming. The physical presence of the researcher can also be intimidating to some respondents, and resulting data can be consciously or subconsciously skewed in the direction of socially desirable answers. They also require a high level of skill on the part of the interviewer to avoid some of the pitfalls outlined.

- The time consuming nature of interviews means that sample size is frequently smaller than that possible with questionnaires.

CHAPTER TEN

Observation

In the last two chapters questionnaires and interviews have been described as methods which try to establish what people do and think by asking them directly. One of the major shortcomings of these two methods is that we have to assume that what people say is what they do. Observation differs in that it collects information first hand based on what people are seen to do by the researcher.

Although it has been suggested that in nursing, observation is not a method that enjoys great popularity (Porter, 1996), there is now an increasing number of midwifery studies that have used this approach, especially in its qualitative form (Kirkham, 1989; Laryea, 1989; Hunt and Symonds, 1995; Davies, 1996).

In this chapter the reasons for using observation will be examined along with its advantages and disadvantages. Two approaches to observation will be highlighted. Firstly, checklist observation will be briefly mentioned and then secondly, qualitative approaches to observation will be outlined in more detail. One of the main aims of the chapter is to demonstrate that there is more to observation than meets the eye!

What is observation?

We are observing the world around us all the time, so what is the difference between 'looking' and 'observing' in a research sense. One of the clearest attempts to differentiate these two terms is provided by Brink and Wood (1994). They suggest that observation stops being a normal part of everyday life and becomes a research method when it is systematically planned and recorded and where both observations and recordings are assessed in terms of their validity and reliability.

LoBiondo-Wood and Haber (1994) define observation as watching with a trained eye for specific events. They suggest that the characteristics of observation include:

* A striving for objectivity
* An attempt to answer a specific research question
* A systematic approach to the activity
* A specific criteria of what should be observed
* A specific time period attached to it
* A record of what is observed and a check made on the accuracy of the observations.

In the research sense, observation is a complex activity which attempts to describe events from the real world. It can be defined as the collection of data which are visible to visual sensors, whether that consists of the researcher's eyes or the use of video.

The nature of the observation can vary, depending on the amount of structure used to record the data. At one extreme is the highly structured observation checklist that leads to quantitative data, and at the other extreme there is the less structured narrative description of events that leads to qualitative data.

Why use observation?

Although we can ask people what they do, we may not always get an accurate answer. The reason is not that people may lie, although that is also possible, but people are not always aware of what they do. In addition, actions can be carried out at a subconscious level and are difficult to explain verbally or write down. Explaining how to tie a shoelace over the phone is an example of this. In many circumstances the best way to find out *how* someone does something is to watch them.

Hardy and Mulhall (1994) suggest that a great advantage of observation is that it enables a researcher to 'get behind' the surface of events and behaviours to reveal the rich complexity of life and activities. This is supported by Holloway and Wheeler (1996) who believe that it is less disruptive and more unobtrusive than interviewing.

Checklist observation

In observations using a written checklist, the researcher lists the kinds of activities they are observing, and then places a tick along side that element each time it is observed. For instance, a checklist of times in an antenatal class a midwife asks those present a direct question as a way of gaining involvement. The results are usually presented numerically, in the form of quantitative data.

Brink and Wood (1994) suggest that the desired behaviours for checklist observation must be explicitly defined so that there is no question in the mind of the observer as to whether or not they occur. In other words clear concept definitions must be developed at the start of the study to ensure the accuracy of the recording.

As events and activities unfold so quickly, there is a limit to the number of different elements the researcher can observe at the same time. Care has to be taken to avoid the checklist becoming too complex. For example, it may not be possible to accurately record the type, duration and form of touch between a midwife and woman in labour, as well as collect duration of eye contact, and non-verbal forms of interaction.

Not only should the number of elements be considered in the checklist, but also the form of recording must be simplified to enable speed and accuracy. Simple ticks or crosses are the best form of recording items. Before using a checklist the researcher should thoroughly practice with a pilot study. This may suggest ways of reducing the complexity of the list, as well as providing the researcher with an opportunity to develop the skill of observing and recording at the same time.

The limitation of an observational checklist is the depth of information that can be achieved, and the limited complexity of interactions that can be accurately observed. This type of approach is also restricted to predicted behaviour, and does not cope well with unexpected activities not included on the checklist. This means it is easy to miss certain forms of behaviour because they have not been anticipated (Brink and Wood, 1994).

Participant and non-participant observation

The more unstructured approach to observation consists of the researcher undertaking data collection either as a participant or non-participant observer, or some variation in between. Holloway and Wheeler (1996) suggest that qualitative researchers generally use participant observation, which they describe as a situation where the social reality of the people observed is examined. This research approach was first developed by anthropologists and sociologists who became part of the culture they studied. Observation allowed them to examine the actions and interactions of people in their natural social context, 'in the field'.

The classic typology of roles an observer may adopt when carrying out data collection was developed by Gold (1958) cited in Holloway and Wheeler (1996). This can be seen in Box 10.1. The different roles vary in the extent to which the researcher becomes directly involved with those observed, and the extent to which the observed are aware that they are being watched.

- **Complete participant**
  The researcher is part of the setting and carries out covert observation as an 'insider'.

- **Participant as observer**
  Observation is overt and is carried out by the researcher who is an insider or has negotiated access to work alongside those in the setting and observe.

- **Observer as participant**
  In this situation the researcher is in the setting but does not have any real involvement with the activities that take place there, the emphasis is on the observation which is overt.

- **Complete observer**
  Here the researcher is at a distance from the setting and what goes on there, and is unnoticed by those who are the subject of the research. Although this can take place unobtrusively from a close vantage point in the setting, such as in a reception area, it is usually applied to a two-way mirror situation, or video link (based on Holloway and Wheeler, 1996)

Box 10.1: Gold's typology of observer role

There are few examples of the complete participant role being adopted in midwifery. An illustration provided by Phillips (1996) is a midwife who joins an early pregnancy class as a client with the intentions of observing what goes on and does not reveal she is both a midwife and researcher. Phillips rightly raises the ethical problems of this kind of deception, although it can be seen that once the identity and purpose of the observer is known, the accuracy of the data obtained may be altered as those involved know that everything is being 'recorded'.

Perhaps one of the most frequently used roles is that of observer as participant. This is where interaction takes place with those who are being observed, and the role of researcher is clearly visible and agreed. A good example is provided by Davies (1996) where the aim of her study was:

> 'to examine the differences and similarities between nursing and midwifery through the eyes of a set of student midwives, and to understand ways in which they attempted to "make sense" of their new world.'

This study illustrates the ethnographic approach to qualitative research where the culture and social world of an identified group are explored by the researcher. In this particular study, the role of the researcher as observer is made clear to the students who gave their permission to be observed. The study involved the researcher in attending lectures and informal activities such as coffee and lunch breaks. The intention of such a study is not to see such activities as a researcher, but to see them through the eyes of those in the setting.

A further example of an ethnographic study is provided by Hunt and Symonds (1995) where Hunt explored the culture of two maternity units over a six month period. The aim of the study was to understand the culture, work practices and strategies of midwives. As with most ethnographic studies the interpretation of the role of observer was not static. Hunt appears to take on the role at times of participant as observer. This can be seen in the following passage.

> 'The maternity unit was frequently very busy and the staff seemed happy to cast me in the role of someone who was an additional pair of hands with some inquisitive and quirky habits (note-taking, etc.)... I was on the outside and on the inside at the same time, and never really "at home". The role is somewhere between stranger and friend.'

Both these studies have much in common, and illustrate the richness of data developed through ethnographic studies. They contrast clearly with checklist observational studies in that the researcher is interested in more in-depth information that does not necessarily follow a clearly anticipated path. There is also a great emphasis on discovering the form of behaviour found in natural settings, such as a labour ward, or department of midwifery studies.

Perhaps in no other form of data collection does the researcher have to consider so carefully their role as researcher, as they play a total and often very visible role within the setting. Hunt (Hunt and Symonds, 1995) for instance at one point has to consider whether she will answer the phone on the ward when it rings. She initially decides not to as this may involve her too much in changing what would have taken place if she had not been there. There is also the danger that performing one activity will adversely affect the role of observer, so for instance she comments:

> 'I did not feel I was capable of being a full-time ethnographer and full-time telephonist.'

Both Hunt and Davies plan carefully the clothes they will wear as researcher. Hunt decides in the early stages to wear a white coat, and comments that,

> 'For someone in a white coat it appeared that access was unrestricted.'

Later this is abandoned once people in the setting are used to her presence, as she felt there was an element of deception in being mistaken for someone 'medical'.

The same degree of thought is illustrated by Davies (1996) in relation to what she wears in the company of the midwifery students. She describes her decision as follows:

> 'I had been careful to choose something relatively unobtrusive from my wardrobe of formal and informal clothing. A simple blouse and skirt and warm sweater seemed to me to be most appropriate for "fitting in" with the students and not the 'uniform' associated with the 'establishment' (I normally wore a smart suit and blouse when visiting as a professional officer).'

The manner of dress can have a profound effect on the way people may react in a situation to someone as researcher. These are not, therefore, trivial details, but are important elements the researcher has included in an attempt to demonstrate credibility, where there is an attempt to share with the reader the nature of the researcher's presence in the research environment.

Recording in observational studies

This section will concentrate on recording in qualitative observational studies. Checklist designs are easier to imagine, as they consist of columns in which a tick is placed if an activity or event is observed. Qualitative observational methods are more complex, and raise more issues for the researcher.

It is tempting to think of observation as simply watching what is happening and only using the sense of sight as the method of collection data. This is far from accurate. Streubert and Carpenter (1995) point out that observation is not intended to mean merely a 'looking at' on the part of the researcher. They stress that observation entails looking, listening, asking questions and collecting artefacts. This last term means including objects which people make or use. In ethnographic studies it frequently takes the form of diaries which subjects may be asked to keep, as in the case of Davies (1996) where she asked the students to keep a diary of their thoughts and experiences.

The major form of recording observations in qualitative studies usually takes the form of field notes. These are narrative accounts of events and situations and can be made while activities are in progress, or they can be written up some time later. DePoy and Gitlin (1994) point out that each alternative has its advantages. Recording while watching, they suggest, may call attention to the observer, however, where notes are written up later there is a greater dependency on the accuracy of memory.

Davies (1996) reveals her strategy for recording field notes, along with some of the problems she encountered as follows:

> 'I kept detailed field notes, which was relatively easy to accomplish in an unobtrusive fashion during classroom activities, but less so during the coffee and lunch breaks and clinical sessions. I recorded the unsolicited interviews as soon after the event as possible. Sometimes I even made notes quickly in the toilet until I discovered Sian and Denise often waited for me, chatting at the washbasins before leaving.'

A similar strategy is used by Hunt (Hunt and Symonds, 1995) and illustrates the amount of data generated in ethnographic studies. Again in the following description the aim is to allow the reader to feel as though they are in the setting and can follow the way in which the data is generated. Hunt describes her recording activities as follows:

> 'My data collection took a variety of forms. The main activity was the production of field notes. During the visit I would use my notebook to record headings and key phrases that would help me in the recording. I also used the dictaphone, usually in the toilet or store cupboard, to record key phrases and prompts. After each visit, when I returned home, I would write detailed field notes on the events of that visit. These were initially filed in date order. The field notes would include details of events and accounts of conversations. Much of the time was spent observing and informal interviewing those who had emerged as key informants. These interviews were unstructured and in the early days I recorded as much as possible of what was said, how it was said, to whom and on what occasions. The field notes also include lengthy descriptions of the labour ward, the office, the admission room, etc.'

These two descriptions provide a comprehensive account of how recording is achieved in a qualitative observational study. It is worth considering that since these two studies took place the availability of 'palm-top' word processors may make the activity slightly easier, but would still draw attention to the procedure.

Advantages

In many situations observation is the most appropriate way of collecting research data as the researcher is able to see what actually happens, and does not depend on reports that may be distorted by memory or perception. In checklist studies the frequency of events can be quantified, and relationships and correlation can be established.

It is in the area of qualitative research that observation can be particularly appropriate to midwifery research. This is especially true where an attempt is made to see things from the point of view of those receiving care (Rees, 1996). Morse and Field (1996) suggest that observation adds breadth to research and provides answers to contextual questions that cannot be answered by interview alone. The important point is that as observation takes place in a natural setting, it can provide an accurate picture of what actually happens. It can also take into account quite a large canvass of activity in the form of a description of say a delivery spread over a long time period.

The works of Kirkham (1989) and Hunt (Hunt and Symonds, 1995) are two good examples of observational studies where the environment of midwifery activities is clearly described in a way that has a familiar realism attached to it. Each, however, provides insights that may go unnoticed by those used to working in those particular areas as they have become 'unremarkable' occurrences.

Qualitative observation also provides flexibility, in that the focus of attention can change as a result of early observations. Barker (1996) argues that the more unstructured the method the more likely it is to allow a deeper insight into the 'workings' of the research setting. He criticises the more structured approaches to data collection, on the grounds that they are mechanistic, and produce only superficial, if not artificial accounts of the research setting.

Observational studies are not frequently found in midwifery although they clearly have a lot to offer in gaining answers to questions that are not amenable to other forms of data collection. As with interviews, they can be used in both a quantitative and qualitative approach, and appear to be eminently suitable for midwifery research either as a single method or in conjunction with other forms of data collection.

Problems in observation

Despite the positive aspects of this method, there are a number of pitfalls that need to be highlighted. Ethical problems are a major concern for the qualitative researcher, especially where covert observation is being used. The issue is one of observing individuals who have not given their permission to be included in a study. This goes against the basic principles of informed consent discussed in Chapter 7.

However, one of the difficulties in observation is the problem of reactivity when people who are told what is being observed may change their normal behaviour as a consequence. Take, for instance, the example given in Chapter 7 of observing student midwives hand-washing techniques and imagine indicating to a student that their technique is about to be observed. The result may be surprisingly good. The observer is likely to be involved in very lengthy observations but probably these would be far from a true picture.

Although LoBiondo-Wood and Haber (1994) agree that observing subjects without their knowledge violates the principle of informed consent, they suggest that sometimes there is no other way to collect such data, and where the data collected is unlikely to have negative consequences for the subject, the disadvantages of the study may be outweighed by the advantages.

A more acceptable answer may be to avoid open deceit by saying, in the case of the student midwife, that routine practices are to be observed, and for data collections to include other activities rather than simply hand washing.

The question of ethics is also raised in situations where the observer sees an activity that may put individuals at risk, or is an unprofessional act carried out by a member of staff (Morse and Field, 1996). Although the researcher tries to maintain a confidential relationship with subjects, in certain circumstances it is not possible to honour this. One example would be where the observer has a public duty to disclose information as in the case of observing something unlawful or which may potentially put a child at risk (Dimond, 1994). A second example would be where an observed activity relates to a breach of the code of professional practice, for example where the activity of another midwife was judged to be unsafe or putting health at risk (UKCC, 1994). In both these examples the researcher is obliged to report these situations, and must abandon the researcher hat for that of the midwife (see Chapter 7 for a discussion of these issues).

From a practical point of view, observation is a very time consuming, and therefore expensive method (Morse and Field, 1996). It also requires a great deal of interpersonal skills on the part of the observer, who should have training and experience with this method. Where more than one person is involved with the data gathering, there is also the problem of inter-observer reliability. This concerns the extent to which different observers select, interpret and record events in different ways.

One of the most obvious problems already referred to is that of reactivity (Morse and Field, 1996), that is, the extent to which the observer influences the activities of those observed. Kirkham (1989) draws attention to this in her work which looked at information giving between midwives and labouring women:

> 'Inevitably, my presence affected what I observed. With midwives this initially had the effect of putting them on their best behaviour. I was quite happy with this as I wanted to know what behaviour these midwives saw as "best" I discounted the observations of my first few hours where conversation was full of effusive "pleases", "thank yous" and "excuse me's".'

This seems an inevitable feature of observations made in the early stages of a study, or in early interactions with individuals. A similar situation is recorded by Hunt (Hunt and Symonds, 1995):

> 'During the early fieldwork stages (the first two or three weeks) it was clear that the staff were making a very special effort to be good communicators. One midwife asked if I would tape her as she encouraged or coached a woman in the second stage of labour. It was an outstanding, energetic performance, worthy of its tape-recording and the language will be familiar to many midwives... The performance seemed to call for an applause and the midwife smiled and seemed almost to bow at the end. She asked if that was what my research was all about. She explained she thought she was a good communicator and I should put this in my research. I promised I would.'

Both these extracts demonstrate the issue of validity. The observer has to consider the extent to which the data is a true picture of what is going on. The ironic tone of both authors' descriptions indicates that it is usually clear to the researcher when observations are not a true reflection of activities.

This challenge to both the reliability of the method, and validity of the results is reduced where the observation is spread over a longer time period where people relax more into their usual way of behaving.

Phillips (1996), drawing on the work of Gans (1982), points out that a further problem is the way the researcher will tend to like certain people in the study, and feel less comfortable with others. This can result in a 'gravitation' towards certain people and an avoidance of others, which may influence the recording process. The best that the researcher can do is to be aware of this through their analysis of the field notes, and attempt to redress the balance. The opposite of this is also true; some people in an observational study will like the researcher, and be willing to spend time with them, and be 'honest' with them. Others, for whatever reason, will feel less positive towards the researcher and will be less of a source of accurate observational and interview material. This situation is not easy to deal with as frequently the researcher is unaware of it.

A further problem for the midwife researcher is the difficulty of being able to stand back from the familiar taken-for-granted routine of the maternity setting, and ask 'why?' In anthropological terms, this is called establishing 'cultural strangeness' where the aim is to see things from an outsiders' point of view.

The longer the researcher is in the field, however, the greater the danger of what is referred to as 'going native'. This term also comes from anthropological studies where, over an extended period of observing tribes, the researcher would become so at home with the new culture that they stop seeing activities and customs as 'strange' or noteworthy. In qualitative research it refers to the researcher becoming over-familiar with the research setting and no longer noticing the kind of elements that need to be included in the observations (Morse and Field, 1996).

A major problem for the researcher is one of selectivity. It is not possible to observe everything that is going on, or see things from every angle, decisions have to be made on where the observer will place themselves, and what they will attempt to observe. This will inevitably lead to some things being observed and others left out. In the same way, it is not possible to record everything, and some details will be omitted (Brink and Wood, 1994).

In some situations there is also the possibility of misinterpreting what is going on. This is particularly true when observing a long established relationship where subtle patterns of communication styles have been developed and understood between people. These can appear strange or alien to the observer. The difference between cajoling someone to do something and apparently being hostile or unsympathetic can be easily misinterpreted by the researcher unaware of the usual pattern of conversation between people.

Observer bias is a further concern, where the researcher may be inclined to look out for certain activities and ignore others that do not fit in with their views or expectations.

Where each period of observation is lengthy, *observer drift* can also be a problem, where the observer loses concentration, and finds themselves thinking of other things, and losing awareness of what is happening. In some situations, time sampling is carried out so that the day is broken down into shorter segments, and the researcher attempts to sample across all the time periods. This allows the researcher to remain relatively fresh throughout the period of observation. Where the researcher is concentrating on events, such as a delivery, this is not always a viable alternative, and an awareness of the danger of observer drift is the only precaution possible.

This range of possible pitfalls illustrates the complexity of this method. A number of excellent examples of qualitative research using observation now exist in midwifery, all of which help the novice researcher to be aware of the problems.

Conducting research

As with each of the methods covered so far, the researcher must ensure that observation is the appropriate method for the study terms of reference. In situations where self reports may be inaccurate, or where there is a need to consider a total process or situation, then observation may be best method to employ.

The decision on which type of observation should be selected is based on the nature of the research question. Where the question relates to a quantification of results, such as 'how often' or 'how much', or where the question is related to establishing whether something happens or not and with what frequency, a checklist design will be called for. This will take the form of a structured sheet which looks like a spread sheet or grid, to allow ease of completion in the form of ticks, code numbers, or letters.

Where the research question does not imply a quantitative approach, but is more concerned with developing a broad understanding of how people act in natural setting, as in an ethnographic study, then a participant, or non-participant observation study should be designed.

The exact role the researcher will play in this kind of research will require a great deal of thought. The variation in role from participant to non-participant observer should be considered (see Box 10.1). It does not necessarily mean that the researcher will stick to the one role. As Streubert and Carpenter (1995) comment, explicit rules for when to participate and when to observe are not available. The consequences of the different types of researcher role, however, must be considered in relation to their influence on those observed and the effect that this will have on the data gathered.

At an early point the ethical implications of the study need to be considered. Where an ethics committee (LREC) is involved, informed consent, and the issue of possible deception should be addressed in a way that will satisfy the committee that consent has been considered, and harm will be avoided.

There are a large number of skills required of the observer. Phillips (1996), for instance, suggests that the observer needs to have good communication skills and a finely tuned sense of 'balance' to maintain what she refers to as 'that marginal yet crucial position of being at one and the same time both participant and observer'.

Hunt (Hunt and Symonds, 1995) elaborates on the skills required of the ethnographer by saying:

> 'Ethnography makes use of basic skills such as listening, watching, asking questions and the skills of 'sussing out".'

By this she means that the researcher has to try and work out what is going on in a situation without using their own stereotypes and preconceptions. Rather, they should try and see things through the eyes of those observed. In terms of the practical activities concerned, DePoy and Gitlin (1994) list three essential activities of i) watching, ii) listening and iii) recording.

This last point raises the issue of what to record, and how. It is important in observation to have clear concept definitions for the items that will be recorded. This is true of checklist observation, as well as qualitative observational approaches.

Hunt (Hunt and Symonds, 1995) provides a useful checklist of what to observe in ethnographic studies by drawing on the seminal work of Spradley (1980) (see Box 10.2).

Space	physical place or places
Actors	the people involved
Activity	set of related acts that people do
Objects	the physical things that are present
Acts	single actions that people do
Events	a set of related activities that people carry out
Time	the sequencing that takes place over time
Goal	the things people are trying to accomplish
Feelings	the emotions felt and expressed

Box 10.2: What to observe

(Source: Spradley 1980, cited by Hunt and Symonds 1995.)

The form of recording will depend on the extent to which contemporary recording may disrupt the flow of activities being observed. The main alternatives will be note taking at the time or some time later, or the use of a dictaphone or tape recorder. DePoy and Gitlin (1994) make the following useful suggestion regarding how the observer should go about recording field notes:

> 'It is often helpful to think of yourself as a video camera and to record what the video camera would see as it scans the boundaries of the research. This technique reminds the researcher that description, not interpretation, is the first step in participant observation.'

The exact details of what is recorded will change during the course of observation. Early notes may be very broad, and will try to establish some ideas of the kind of pattern of activity taking place. They will then become more focused depending on earlier observations, and the questions arising from the field notes. An idea of the content of early field notes is provided by Hunt (Hunt and Symonds, 1995) as follows:

> 'The field notes were generally descriptive accounts of events observed in the field. Direct quotations were included whenever possible as were descriptions of such aspects as the tone of voice and the body language of the contributor. The field notes also included sketches of some aspects of the environment and maps to remind me of the layout of the unit.'

The analysis stage of this kind of data is a very sophisticated activity. As with the analysis of quantitative data, advice and help should be sought from those with experience of this type of data.

In presenting the qualitative report or article, the structure is very different from that of a quantitative report or article. Some of the sources of work referred to in this chapter should be considered as a guide for writing the report in order to do full justice to the information collected.

Critiquing research

In critiquing observational research articles, we have to decide whether this was a suitable method to answer the research question. It is important to determine what the researcher was observing and how. In both checklist and qualitative approaches, does the researcher give a clear concept definition for the items being observed?

Was the study approved by an ethics committee? Was the research overt or covert, that is were people aware that they were being observed or not? Was permission sought from subjects where it was overt? Where permission was not sought, does the researcher provide a convincing justification for not securing this?

Where the researcher is active in the research setting, we must consider the extent to which they may have had an influence on the people and events observed. What did the researcher do to try to minimize the reactive effect on subjects? In good qualitative studies we should expect the researcher to provide a clear description of how they presented themselves in the setting in terms of dress, and behaviour.

The role the researcher decided to play is important in deciding the extent to which people in the setting may have reacted to them. Which of the possible roles did the researcher select, and does this appear to have been a good choice? Did the researcher appear to display any bias, emotions, prejudices in their dealings with those observed which may have influenced the quality of the data collected? Does the researcher appear to gravitate towards certain people in the study, and avoid others? In other words has there been a bias in who was observed which may have produced untypical results?

Where more than one observer was responsible for the data collection, what checks were there that inter-observer reliability was achieved? Even where there is only one observer, it is important to establish if any training was received or a pilot study undertaken. An excellent example is set by Davies (1996) who took her research supervisor to her pilot study of a group of students attending a study day. She then compared her field notes with those of the experienced supervisor.

Has the researcher included other methods of data collections such as structured or unstructured interviews, or the use of diaries, or other form of documentary methods? Either with observation alone or with other methods, the researcher using a qualitative approach should have produced, 'thick' or 'rich' data (Hardy and Mulhall, 1994). Does this enhance credibility so it almost feels as if you are there?

When it comes to analysis, does the researcher leave a decision trail so that you can audit the way they have moved through the data collection to the establishment of the categories used to present the findings? Overall, does the researcher convince you that they have tried to be as rigorous as possible throughout the study?

KEY POINTS

- Observation can be used to produce quantitative or qualitative data.

- Although it is not used as often as some of the other methods, it can play an important part in answering important questions in an holistic and woman centred way.

- In observation the main issue is the extent to which the researcher can control the influence of their presence on what is observed.

- There are a large number of strategies which must be decided by the researcher such as the nature of the role they will play, the amount of interaction they will have with those observed, the method of recording, the extent of recording, and the method of analysis.

- The time period needed for some studies makes this a costly method of collecting data and one that requires a large amount of personal skills, as well as research expertise. The benefits of such an approach, however, are considerable.

CHAPTER ELEVEN

Experiments

Experimental design has established itself as the most widely recognized, and respected, approach to research within the health service. In medicine the most popular form of the experiment is the randomized control trial (RCT). This method of collecting research data has become so powerful in determining the effectiveness of treatments, that it is used by some as a measure against which all other methods are compared.

The basic goal of the experiment is to produce evidence of the existence of a cause and effect relationship between two variables. These are the independent variable (the cause), and the dependent variable (the effect). Such studies usually take the form of a comparison between an experimental and control group.

As many clinical procedures in maternity care are influenced by both midwifery and obstetric experimental research, it is crucial that the midwife is able to evaluate such studies to ensure that they are not accepted without question. The presentation of such studies tends to be based very much on statistical analysis, and this can form a barrier to comprehension. Midwives can become depowered if they do not understand the basis on which clinical trails are carried out, and how to interpret the findings. Similarly, midwives should know how to carry out trials alone, or as an informed partner in multidisciplinary trails.

The purpose of this chapter is to consider the basic principles of the experiment, to recognize their strengths, as well as their limitations, and to outline some of the alternative forms they take.

Why are experiments special?

Experiments are sometimes regarded as not only different from other broad research approaches such as surveys, but are thought to have a higher status. Talbot (1995), for example, points out that the true experimental design is considered to be the classic form of research. Oakley (1992) also notes that the Randomized Control Trial (RCT) has been characterized within medicine and health care research generally as 'the most scientifically valid method' of research.

More recently Hicks (1996), in her text book on midwifery research, concentrates almost exclusively on the experimental approach. Why do experimental designs have such a high status, especially amongst the medical community? The answer lies in what they can achieve and the characteristics they possess.

Firstly, in terms of what they can achieve, Burnard and Morrison (1994) note that experimental research attempts to establish 'laws'. The ability to say reasonably accurately that one thing can cause something else is a very potent characteristic that allows predictions to be made. This is achieved through their ability to eliminate the influence of other factors that may affect the results of a study (Talbot, 1995). The extent to which a causal link has been demonstrated is through the calculation of the extent to which the results could have happened by chance. This is indicated by the 'p' value which is frequently to be found under a table of results or in the text of a research article (see Box 11.1).

Probability values indicate the extent to which the difference in the results between two groups could have happened by chance. The 'p' means 'probability'. This is interpreted in terms of how many times out of a hundred, or even a thousand, the difference between two groups of data could happen purely by chance.

The value of 'p' is expressed as a decimal, and has to be converted to a fraction to establish the element of chance. Take the example of p = 0.05. We first of all convert 0.05 to a fraction by drawing a line underneath the figure; put a '1' underneath the decimal point, and a '0' for every figure after it. So 0.05 becomes 5/100. In other words the likelihood of the difference between the two groups of data happening purely by chance is 5 in 100 times.

This is regarded as the minimum value that may suggest a relationship between the dependent and independent variable. Notice that there is a margin of error. It does not mean that one thing definitely causes the other; the results would have happened purely by chance five in a hundred times. This means that for 95 per cent of the time you can be satisfied that a cause and effect relationship does exist. This is sometimes referred to as the 95 per cent confidence level. In other words we are 95 per cent confident that there is a relationship between the independent and dependent variable.

The most frequently used values to indicate probability are as follows:

p value	probability of difference happening by chance
0.05	5 in 100
0.01	1 in 100
0.001	1 in 1000
NS	non-significant (i.e. the probability that chance is responsible for the result is so large that a 'p' value is not used).

It is recommended that you consult a statistics book such as Clegg (1982) for more information.

Box 11.1: Probability values

Characteristics of experimental design

What are the essential features of an experiment? According to Mulhall (1994), the following should be evident:

- Manipulation of an independent variable
- Measurement of the impact of the independent variable on the dependent variable
- Minimizing, or accounting for, the effects of factors other than the independent variable on the dependent variable
- Identification of a causal relationship between an independent and dependent variable.

Other writers suggest that an experiment can be identified by the presence of the following three features:

- Manipulation
- Control
- Randomization.

These characteristics were first suggested by Campbell and Stanley (1963) and are now taken as the authoritative elements of experimental design. Each of these is discussed below.

Manipulation

According to Mulhall (1994), manipulation is the hallmark of the experimental design, and consists of being able to make the independent variable present in one group, and not the other in a study. Hicks (1996) suggests that the simplest way to find out whether a relationship exists between two variables is to alter one and see what difference it makes to the other. It is the ability to apply and withhold the independent variable that is unique to the true experiment, and enables the researcher to suggest that the outcome is due to the independent variable.

Control

Here, the researcher must try to reduce the possible effect of other independent variables on the outcome. This means that the experimenter must have the ability to not only control the independent variable but also other elements within the experimental setting that might make a difference to the outcome. For example, they must be able to choose who takes part in the study, or at least ensure that every one in the study has an equal chance of being in the experimental group (random allocation). If this is achieved then the researcher can say that they have controlled for extraneous factors which may influence the dependent variable.

It is the researcher's ability to achieve maximum control that illustrates the degree of rigour in the study. Burns and Grove (1995) point out that control includes the way any interventions are provided. All procedures must be applied in exactly the same way to each individual. Burns and Grove (1995) also suggest that control extends to the measurements within the study. The measuring instrument should be accurate and consistent, and where more than one person is involved in the measurement, the researcher should ensure that everyone is measuring in the same way.

Randomization

Randomization may apply to both the sampling procedure and the allocation of individuals to control or intervention groups (Mulhall, 1994). Random sampling occurs when every member of a study population (all those with the relevant characteristics) has an equal chance of being included in the sample. In many studies this is not easy to achieve as individuals must first agree to take part in a clinical study. In most cases randomization refers to random assignment or allocation. This is the process of placing subjects who have agreed to take part in a study in either the experimental or control group in a random manner. In other words, an individual entering the study should have an equal chance of receiving the treatment or intervention. The ability to achieve this depends on those entering the study being happy to accept 'pot luck' in relation to the type of care or procedure they will receive (Alexander, 1995).

The implication of not using random allocation is emphasized by De Poy and Gitlin (1994) who say that without it the investigator is at risk of developing groups that initially differed from each other. This would make it impossible to rule out the influence of other factors, or independent variables, on the results and make generalizations very difficult.

Where randomization has been achieved it reduces the opportunity for researcher bias. This is because the researcher is unable to influence the results by carefully choosing the experimental group on the basis of their possession of factors that will favour the hypothesis (Oakley, 1992). Randomization also ensures that additional factors that may also influence the results are evenly distributed between the two groups. In other words, randomization should allow the researcher to compare like with like.

The existence of a comparison group which does not receive the independent variable is crucial to experimental design. De Poy and Gitlin (1994) suggest that the role of the control group is to establish what the outcome would be without the influence of the experimental variable. The control group theoretically remains the same over the experimental period, that is at the pre-test and post-test period. This allows the investigator to examine what has variously been referred to as the 'attention factor', the 'Hawthorne effect' or the 'halo effect'. These terms all relate to the phenomena where individuals may experience change simply through participation in a study.

In some studies there may not be a separate group who form the control. One group can receive two interventions, for example a conventional approach and then an experimental approach. In this way individuals act as their own control. It is also possible for two separate groups to receive two interventions, but in a different order. Here again they are acting as their own controls in that they receive both interventions and rule out the possibility that any differences are the results of characteristics which vary in the two groups. This kind of approach is referred to as a *cross-over study*.

The hypothesis

Brink and Wood (1994) categorize the experiment as a level 3 research question. To achieve this level they suggest that the researcher should be able to predict what will happen (have a hypothesis), and provide a theory based on previous research findings to explain it. One of the chief purposes of the experiment is to test a hypothesis and so establish causality. The hypothesis must be stated by the researcher at the start of the study. This can take two forms; the *scientific hypothesis* and the *null-hypothesis*. The scientific hypothesis states the prediction that the researcher is making in relation to the difference in outcome between the two groups. It usually contains words such as 'more than' or 'less than', whereas the null-hypothesis predicts that there will be no difference between the two groups (see Chapter 6).

For those unfamiliar with hypotheses, it is not always easy to work out which is the dependent and which is the independent variable in the statement. Hick (1996) suggests one way of working this out is to say what depends on what? The thing that depends on something else is the dependent variable. An alternative method is to identify which comes first chronologically and which comes last. The item that comes last is the dependent variable (the effect), and the item that comes first is the independent variable (the cause). Box 11.2 provides some examples of hypotheses and illustrates the dependent and independent variables in each case.

- Women with inverted or non-protractile nipples, when advised to use breast shells and/or Hoffman's exercises *(independent variable)* would be more likely to succeed with breastfeeding until six weeks postnatally *(dependent variable)* than if no such intervention had taken place (Alexander et al., 1992).

- The effects of the social support intervention *(independent variable)* on a variety of pre-specified health outcomes *(dependent variables)* would favour mothers and babies allocated to the intervention group (Oakley, 1994).

- The treatment of women under 37 weeks pregnant with idiopathic preterm labour or prelabour rupture of the membranes with oral broad-spectrum antibiotics (Augmentin and erythromycin), *(independent variable)* reduces the neonatal morbidity associated with preterm birth *(dependent variable)* (Kenyon and Taylor, 1995).

- The way in which care is given by midwives during the postnatal period *(independent variable)* will influence the emotional response of women to the changes which follow the birth of a child *(dependent variable)* (Ball, 1989).

Box 11.2: Examples of scientific hypotheses

Types of experiments

Medical research is frequently associated with the term randomized control trial (RCT). Although treated as synonymous with 'scientific research design', this design is only just over fifty years old. Oakley (1992) traces its origins to the work of the Medical Research Council (MRC) and the introductions of streptomycin as a treatment for TB. Studies had just been completed on animals that suggested it may be an effective cure for the disease. The animals subjected to the test were guinea pigs, hence the expression 'to be a guinea pig' meaning the subject of an experiment. At the time there was a shortage of the new drug streptomycin, and a large number of people with TB. The Medical Research Council were permitted to allocate the drug to people on the basis of selection using a table of random numbers in an attempt to confirm the effectiveness of the drug. This was the first documented use of the randomized control trial.

Experimental design can take a number of alternative forms. The classic writers on the subject, Campbell and Stanley (1963), suggest that there are three main variations:

- The pre-test-post-test control group
- The post-test only
- The Solomon four design.

The pre-test post-test group is perhaps the most well known design where subjects are randomly allocated to the experimental or control group. Both groups are observed prior to any intervention, and this acts as a base-line measurement. At this point any important differences between the two groups should be minimal. In the intervention phase, the experimental group will receive the new procedure, or treatment variable, while the control group is either treated in the usual way or does not receive treatment (although they may receive a placebo). Both groups are then retested, and any difference in measurements between the two groups are subjected to statistical analysis through the use of inferential statistics which calculate the possibility that the difference could be a chance variation, and not the result of the test procedure (Fig. 11.1).

This method can be carried out using two different groups measured over the same time period, or, as indicated earlier, a single group can be used which receives first one variable and then another. In this way they act as their own controls. This has the advantage that it reduces the possibility that those in the control group are not quite comparable with the experimental group. Hicks (1996) calls this first approach of two different groups unrelated, between, or different subject design, and calls the second example a related, within or same subject design. It is worth considering that where there is only one group receiving first one intervention then another, there can be a 'carry-over' effect, in that any benefits from the first variable may still influence the individual once exposed to the second variable. To reduce this possibility the order in which individuals are exposed to each procedure is sometimes randomized.

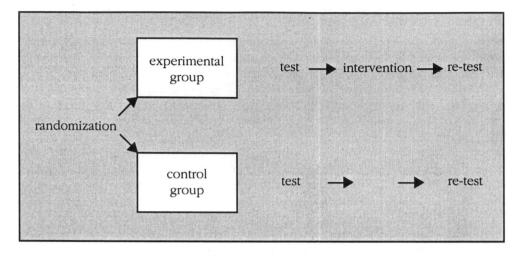

Fig. 11.1: The pre-test, post-test design

Post-test only design

A problem with the pre-test-post-test design is that measuring the groups before treatment is not always possible. There is also the problem that the first measurement may sensitize the subjects in such a way that they perform better on the second occasion because of the experience gained during the first measurement. The post-test only design (Fig. 11.2) is an attempt to reduce this familiarity effect by only measuring the variables at the end of the experimental period. The limitation of this design is that it is not possible to say whether the two groups were similar at the start of the study. The difference in measurement could have been due to characteristics existing within the groups.

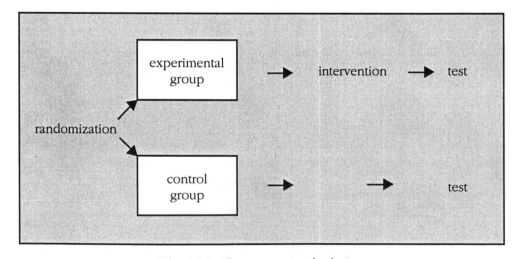

Fig. 11.2: The post-test only design

Solomon four design

In order to overcome the disadvantages of both the previous examples, the Solomon four group design has been developed. As can be seen from Figure 11.3, this is really a combination of both the previous designs. This means that as well as being able to eliminate the disadvantage of an after-only design, the effect of pre-testing can be scrutinized.

The immediate problem is one of getting a sufficient number of subjects for all four groups. In addition, the possibility of some people dropping out (subject mortality) is even greater with this number of participants. The researcher may no longer be comparing like with like if the numbers in some of the groups have changed during the study period. This kind of design is very complex to organize and costly. Overall, we can see that this is a large scale design which requires a great deal of time, resources and expertise.

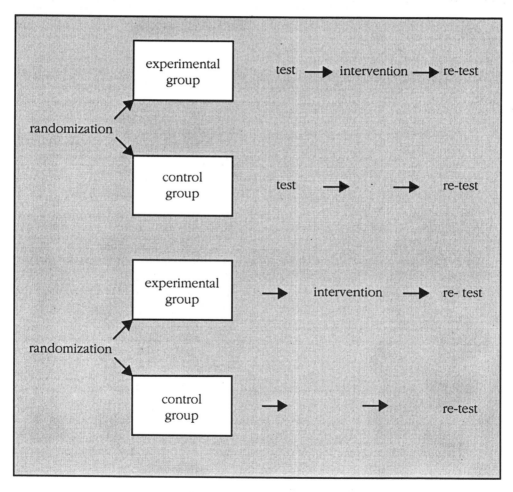

Fig. 11.3: The solomon four-group design

Threats to validity

Although experimental designs are held in high regard, their use does not guarantee accuracy. There are a number of reasons why the results of an experiment may be inaccurate. Campbell and Stanley (1963) provide the best summary of these problems which are usually referred to as the threats to validity. These threats come in two types; those which relate to the experiment itself (internal threats to validity) and those which relate to generalizing the results to other situations (external threats to validity).

Campbell and Stanley (1963) identify a number of problem areas in relation to *internal validity*. Any of the following may result in the researcher incorrectly suggesting they had found a causal relationship between the dependent and independent variable:

- **History (the effect of external events on study outcomes)**
  This relates to situations where it is not the study independent variable that has influenced the outcome, but something outside the study, sometimes referred to as a *confounding variable*. For example, media reports highlighting an issue such as problems related to the contraceptive pill, or publicity given to a celebrity choosing to breastfeed may influence the behaviour, attitude or knowledge of those in a study. The impact of 'historical' events may be mistaken for the result of an intervention applied in a study.

- **Testing (the effect that being observed or tested has on the study outcomes)**
  This refers to the consequence of being tested at one point in time on the results of a later re-test. Undergoing the first test may have made an individual think about issues and influence how they answer later on the re-test. Here, it is the consequence of the first test and not the intervention that has made a difference to the results.

- **Instrumentation (the extent to which the instrument used to gather information in the study is accurate)**
  The consequence of instrumentation is that there may be a problem with the instrument used to collect data changing over time, or the skills or accuracy of the data gatherers may change over time and so different measurements may be produced which is interpreted as due to the independent variable under study.

- **Maturation (the effect of the passage of time on individuals in the sample)**
  This relates to studies that extend over a time period such as pregnancy and early months of motherhood, where normal physical, psychological, and social changes occur to individuals that may be unrelated to the variables in the study. Over time individuals will physically change, adapt, develop new skills, change attitude and so on. It is also possible for maturation changes to occur over shorter periods. Even in the course of a day we can get tired, or develop insights or physical abilities which, if subjected to retesting, may suggest a change due to an intervention rather than a normally occurring event.

- **Regression (a statistical phenomenon)**

  This is a frequently observed situation in statistics where there is a tendency for extreme scores or measurements in a study to regress, or move closer to the mean (average) when repeated testing takes place. This relates to before and after measurements (pre-test/post-test).

- **Mortality (the effect caused by people dropping out of a study before all the measurements have been made)**

  Although an experimental and control group may have been similar at the start of a study, those who decided to pull out of the study may have shared some common characteristic such as age, parity, or have been smokers, etc. Those remaining are no longer quite as similar as those in the other group, so the researcher is no longer comparing like with like.

- **Interactive effects (the extent to which each of these threats interact with sample selection to influence the outcome of a study)**

  In the same way that the above individual threats may influence those in one group rather than another, so the range of influences may be acting on all those selected to form members of the different groups, influencing the results.

External validity considers those factors which limit the extent to which findings can apply to other settings. Although there are not as many threats as with internal validity, the consequences can be just as serious. There are three main threats that need to be considered, and these relate to the people selected for inclusion in the study; the factors relating to what happens within the experiment itself, and the measurements carried out to produce the results.

LoBiondo-Wood and Haber (1994) refer to these as:

- The effects of selection
- Reactive effects
- Effects of testing.

The *effect of selection* relates to the extent to which the characteristics of the sample may not have been truly representative of the population, and so it is unwise to generalize from the results of this particular sample. For instance, in some experiments women from a particular social class, age group, or parity may have been over-represented in the sample. This may have produced results that cannot be applied to all women.

The *reactive effect* is the way in which some people respond to being in an experiment. For example, one woman in the control group in Oakley's (1992) social support study said she felt special because she was part of a study. In an experimental situation some people may react to the experiment in ways which are due to feeling special, or a desire for the experimenter to succeed, and so the results are not really due to the independent variable.

This was found in the American study on motivation that looked at people working in what was known as the Hawthorn plant of an electricity company in Kansas. Although the study was examining the effect of heating and lighting and other environmental factors on output, it was found that whether these factors were raised or lowed, productivity increased. It was realized that it was not the heating or lighting which was affecting the output, but feeling special because they were receiving attention from researchers that influenced their work. This gave rise to the term 'Hawthorn effect', which relates to the reactive effect of being part of a study.

Finally, in relation to *the effect of testing*, if we accept that pretesting knowledge or attitude may influence re-testing, (due to people having an opportunity to reflect on how they feel about the subject of the test), then we have to acknowledge that testing may reduce the extent to which the results of the study can be applied to others. This is because following testing those in the sample are no longer typical of other people, as they have experienced something, or reflected on subjects or values that makes them different from others.

One further problem area relates to the experimenter. Bias may develop where the researcher in their enthusiasm for the study may subconsciously influence people in non-verbal ways, such as positive nods of the head, or smiling when certain answers are given. This source of error has been described as *experimenter bias effect* (Hicks, 1996). Similarly, those in the study may provide answers or try hard to carry out the wishes of the experimenter because they like the individual and want the study to be successful. Their reactions to the procedures may also be affected by their knowledge of whether they are in the experimental or control group.

Attempts to reduce these problems are through the use of *blind* and *double blind* studies. *Blind studies* are where either the person collecting the data, or the subjects in the study, are unaware of:

i)   the hypothesis being tested,
ii)   who is in the experimental or control group.

Often in blind clinical trials the person collecting the measurements, or conducting interviews is not part of the study design team, and is unaware of what the researchers are looking for. In this way they are unable to influence the outcome, even a subconscious level. In a *double blind study* neither the data collector nor the subject is aware of who is in the experimental or control group, or the nature of the hypothesis being tested.

Quasi-experimental and ex post facto designs

Although experimental design is regarded as one of the strongest methods of establishing cause and effect relationships, it is not always possible to use this approach in every situation. The reasons can be practical, in terms of being able to control the effect of other independent variables, or ethical, in that it would not be acceptable to allocate people to an experimental and control group. For example, it would not be ethical to allocate some women to say a water-birth delivery and others a bed delivery, as this would take away choice. Similarly, it would not be possible to randomly allocate women to a smoking or no smoking group to examine the consequence on the fetus.

Where the strict conditions of experiments are not possible, there are a number of near alternatives that can be used. The first is the *quasi-experiment*. This looks very much like an experiment with often an experimental and control group, and with the researcher introducing an intervention. Where it differs is that there is a lack of at least one of the basic elements of the experiment of either control, or randomization. In most cases it tends to be a lack of random allocation to the two groups that is missing. An example would be women on one ward having sessions on relaxation to measure its effect on mood and a positive attitude to coping with life following delivery, and those on a second ward being used as a control without relaxation. This makes it a lot easier to manager as all those in one setting will be receiving the same approach. It also reduces the risk of 'contamination' where individuals may be influenced by what they see happening to those along side them.

Unfortunately, having all those in one setting receiving the intervention, rather than random allocation, will weaken the extent to which we can rule out threats to validity. It could be that there are differences between those in the two groups that could make a difference to the outcome. In this relaxation example, it could be that some women already practice yoga, or meditation, or that there were differences in personalities between women on the two wards.

For these reason quasi-experimental studies are not as convincing as a true experimental design. It is possible to strengthen them as much as possible by taking measurements of both groups prior to the intervention so that we can see the extent to which they are similar and can be accepted as reasonably comparable. In research terms, this approach of two non-randomized groups is referred to as *non-equivalent control group* design.

Ex post facto studies

In quasi experimental design, although randomization was not achieved, the researcher still manipulated the independent variable, exposing the experimental group to the intervention, but not the control group. In some situations, not only is it difficult to carry out randomization, but it can also be difficult to manipulate the independent variable. In this instance the solution is the use of ex post facto studies. This term means that the difference between the two groups in relation to the independent variable has already happened (ex post facto means after the fact). So, for instance, we might be interested in establishing whether going to antenatal classes has some baring on the successful use of birth plans. Again it could be difficult to construct a study and allocate women to the antenatal class attendance group, and others to the antenatal class non-attendance group, as they would be depriving some of the latter access to facilities that they may want, and from which they may gain a wide range of benefits.

An ex post facto study would collect data on women who were judged to have made good use of a birth plan and those who made little use of a birth plan, and try to establish if there was any pattern in which group had the greater number of women who had attended antenatal classes. In this design we are looking for associations that are provided by *correlation*. This statistical process allows us to identify the extent to which factors seem to go together. Unfortunately, we cannot say that one causes the other, only that they appear to be linked. However, this may be satisfactory in providing the basis for midwifery action, or increasing our ability to predict certain events.

One example of an ex post facto study is that by Siney et al (1995) which looked at opiate dependency in pregnancy. This retrospective study compared outcomes in opiate dependent women who were on a methadone programme during their pregnancy and receiving regular antenatal care, and non-drug-misusing women matched by age, parity and postcode. In this situation the drug dependency had already occurred. It would not be possible to allocate women to a drug-dependency group or a non-drug-dependency group, and so an ex post facto approach is as close as we can get to a systematic study of the consequence of this situation.

The strength of both quasi-experimental and ex post facto designs is their practical nature, they are far more feasible and because they avoid some of the ethical issues of experimental designs they are very attractive designs within midwifery.

Conducting research

In deciding to undertake an experimental study, it is important to confirm that this is an appropriate approach. Where the purpose of the study is to determine the existence of a cause and effect situation, then an experimental approach is appropriate. If the purpose is to search for factors that are associated with each other, and not necessarily as part of a cause and effect relationship, a correlation design will be more appropriate.

Once the appropriateness of an experimental design has been established, the researcher should ensure that the three defining factors of an experiment are feasible. These are:

- Manipulation
- Control
- Randomization.

In addition to these, the researcher must consider the ethical elements of the study, particularly in relation to possible harm through an intervention or the withholding of accepted interventions. The research should also avoid raising the expectations of those involved or put them into stressful situations. It is advisable to re-read Chapter 7 on ethics in order to ensure that possible problem areas have been anticipated.

As informed consent is an integral part of experimental approaches, it is a good idea to design a written consent form which those involved in the study will be required to sign, along with an information sheet ready to include with your proposal for the Local Research Ethics Committee (LREC). Examples of these may be available locally from others who have undertaken research; from dissertations in educational libraries, or from the ethics committee itself.

In planning the study, previous research should be examined carefully, with special attention paid to the design. In particular, how did the researchers address the threats to internal and external validity. The literature should also provide clues as to the relevant independent variables to be included, and the additional variables that may confound the results, that is cloud the ability to say that the results have been produced by the independent variable(s) manipulated in this study.

In an experimental study the construction of the hypothesis is a major part of the planning process. This should be a clear statement that includes the dependent and independent variable(s). The form of the hypothesis should be considered in terms of whether it will be *directional*, that is it will predict the results from the experimental group will be higher or lower than the control group (referred to as a *one-tailed hypothesis)*, *non directional*, that is it will suggest there will be a difference without saying whether it will be higher or lower in a particular group, (referred to as a *two-tailed hypothesis* as the results could go either way), or a *null-hypothesis*, where it would be stated that there would be no difference between the two groups.

It is at this stage serious thought should be given to what information will need to be collected to test the hypothesis. This will have to be in a numeric form, and will be subjected to a statistical test. There are a variety of tests, depending on the form of the experiment and the nature of the numeric values. It is at the early design stage that the statistical procedures required should be explored. It is recommended that an appropriate book that includes statistical test is consulted (Hicks, 1996) and help and advice sought from someone who is knowledgeable on statistical techniques.

In order to reduce bias as much as possible, thought needs to be given to who will collect the data. In some instances it may be feasible, as well as highly desirable, to have someone not directly involved with the design of the study collect data blind, that is, without knowing the hypotheses to be tested, and without knowing whether subjects are in the experimental or control group. At the design stage the necessity and method of blinding the subjects should also be considered.

Where data is being collected by several people, steps should be taken to ensure they measure, code, or collect the information in exactly the same way and with the same degree of accuracy (referred to as *inter-rator or inter-observer reliability*). This attention to consistency, and accuracy should extend to any equipment used as part of the study, or any materials such as Likert scales or other form of measurements.

The way the study is carried out must be carefully recorded in sufficient detail so that it can be used by anyone wishing to replicate the study. A pilot study is essential to familiarize yourself with the equipment and the procedure.

When conducting the main study, the safety and welfare of the subjects is paramount. In some instances the decision may have to be made to immediately remove individuals from the study for their own benefit, and transfer them to standard procedures, or treatments. On other occasions, there may be factors that develop during the study that make some people no longer typical within the group, and they may have to be excluded at the analysis stage. For example, Kirkham (1989) removed from her observational study any women for whom she provided direct information, which made them no longer dependent on the midwives providing the care for information in labour. All these factors relate to the rigour of the study.

At the end of an experimental study it is important to base the conclusions only on the results. The statistical tests will provide some answer as to the strength of the relationship between the independent and dependent variables. It is important to recognize that these tests only relate to a statistical relationship between the figures and do not necessarily imply that a real world relationship exists. There is always a margin of error in experimental studies. In addition, the sometimes artificial circumstances and environment make generalizations very difficult. Medicine has always placed a great emphasis on replication studies to ensure that the results of a single study do not influence practice without the corroboration of further studies. It is important that midwifery also recognizes the importance of replication.

Where it is not possible for practical, or ethical reasons to carry out a true experimental design, then the researcher should choose the next appropriate design, such as quasi-experimental or ex post facto approaches. These may play an important part in providing valuable answers for practice. The rigour of these kinds of design is just as important as in experimental design, if not more so, as the evaluation of such studies will start with the view that they are not as strong as experimental design. Clear attempts should therefore be made to reduce the possibility of the results being explained by factors other than the ones being suggested by the researcher.

All the designs in this section depend on a very clear statistical presentation of the results. It is this aspect of research reports that many midwives find most baffling. For this reason the midwifery researcher should explain the statistical procedures used, and clarify their meaning and implications for the reader as clearly as possible.

Critiquing research

Critiquing experimental research can be challenging, mainly because of the reader's unfamiliarity with statistical presentation. Yet a little knowledge and understanding of some of the basic concepts and conventions can clarify the report drastically. The first stage of critiquing is to ensure that the researcher is searching for a cause and effect relationship between an independent and dependent variable. This will usually be evident from the wording of the terms of reference which will suggest the influence of, or relationship between, one variable and another. Experimental research should contain a hypothesis, although sadly, this is not present in all reports.

In reading the details of the conduct of the study the three features of an experiment, manipulation, control and randomization, should be present. If randomization, or control are not present, it may be a quasi-experimental study. If the researcher states the intention is to look for associations or possible relationships, then the study is likely to be a correlation design. Here it will not be possible for the researcher to talk in terms of cause and effect, or dependent and independent variables.

Where the study is clearly experimental, consideration should be given to the ethical component. Was the study approved by an ethics committee, or in the case of an American report an Institutional Review Body (IRB)? To what extent did the subjects in the study clearly give their informed consent? Was it made clear that participation in the study was optional, and it was possible to withdraw at any point? Did the author make an assessment of possible harm, and build in safeguards to discontinue involvement or, through clear exclusion criteria, prevent any vulnerable individuals from entering the study in the first place?

The sample included in the study should be scrutinized in relation to the inclusion and exclusion criteria for those selected for the study. The method of randomization should be considered to ensure that everyone had an equal chance of being selected for the experimental group. A close comparison should then be made of the groups to ensure that they are comparable in those factors that might have made a difference to the results. Remember they should be as similar as possible in all respects apart from the exposure to the independent variable under study.

The researcher should give clear concept and operational definitions for the dependent and independent variables. These should be considered for their adequacy. The type of intervention should be considered carefully in terms of how did the researcher make sure that it was provided in a similar way to everyone? Was there any check on this, such as training for those involved in providing the intervention to ensure consistency? In particular, an assessment should be made of possible inaccuracies in the measurements made following the intervention. Was this a blind or double-blind study? If not, does this lead to any possible weaknesses?

In examining the results section, has the researcher used an appropriate test of significance to test the probability that any differences between groups could have happened by chance? Here the size of the 'p' value is important. In considering the results, to what extent has the researcher taken into account the possible threats to internal and external validity? It is worth considering whether the results could be explained by some other factor besides the independent variable.

Depending on the results, what are the implications for practice? What specific recommendations are made in the report? Whatever the researcher says, it is important to remember the importance of the reliability of the data collection tool(s), the validity of the study in terms of is there evidence that they have measured what they believe they have measured? Are there any biasing factors concerning those selected for the study? And finally, are you satisfied with the rigour with which the researcher conducted the study? Is there a striving for excellence in the way the whole study was put together, and carried out?

Above all, do not simply be impressed by the size of the study, its complexity, or the use of statistics. As with any kind of study it is crucial to challenge the research, and recognize both the lengths the researcher has gone to in order to maintain accuracy, and the limitations of the study, and the implications that these will have for the extent to which you can generalize to your own situation. With all clinical trials it is also wise to look for confirming evidence from replication studies before adopting a system that may have considerable implications for the delivery of services and the health of those concerned.

KEY POINTS

- Experimental designs, particularly in the form of the randomized control trial, have become one of the most respected types of research in the health service. The reason for this relates to the way that drugs and treatments in the past have been carefully tested to rule out as far as possible, other explanations for the results.

- The conduct of such studies can be very complex because they are dependent on the three necessary experimental elements of control, manipulation and randomization. In midwifery, it is not always possible, or desirable, to achieve these elements. Sometimes it would be unethical, or at least drastically reduce women's choice or individual midwife's judgement on what was best in the particular circumstances, if strict experimental protocols were followed.

- There are compromises available in the form of quasi-experimental, ex post facto and correlational designs which, although they do not produce results that are as 'strong' as experimental design, can still influence practice.

- Despite the status given to experimental designs, they do have their limitations. It is not always possible to control for other factors which may explain the results. In addition, it is sometimes an over-simplification to look for one cause for a phenomenon; sometimes there are several.

- One of the necessary elements in this type of design is the use of statistical methods. These identify the influence of chance in explaining the difference in the results between groups. The knowledge required to understand and challenge this form of research is therefore more demanding than some of the other methods. Midwives should not see this as a reason for avoiding this research approach, or reading published work. The effort needed to gain the statistical knowledge and understanding is well worth the reward of being able to confidently use and challenge this method.

CHAPTER TWELVE

Sampling Methods

The outcome of any research project is dependent on both the reliability of the method used, and the type and quality of the sample on whom the results are based. In this chapter the issues relating to who or what is included in the sample, and the alternative methods for choosing the sample will be examined.

First we must clarify the difference between a 'population' and 'sample'. Although these terms appear to be used almost interchangeably, there is a clear difference between them.

The *population* is the total group of people, things or events the researcher is interested in saying something about, e.g. midwives who have a degree or higher qualification, women who have a home delivery etc. DePoy and Gitlin (1994) suggest we think of a population as the complete set of elements that share a common set of characteristics. We can then define a *sample* as a proportion of the population which has been selected to 'stand for' the total group.

There are a number of alternative ways of arriving at a sample The choice will vary depending on whether the research approach can be described as:

- Experimental
- Survey
- Qualitative.

The method of choosing the sample will also be influenced by how far the researcher wants to generalize the findings to the wider population. The more important it is to achieve this, the more complex the sampling strategy used.

Whatever the purpose of the study, the researcher is faced with three vital questions:

- Who or what will make up the sample?
- How are they to be chosen?
- How many will be chosen?

The chapter will illustrate the way in which the researcher attempts to answer these questions.

Why sample?

Why bother to sample in the first place? Surely it must be more accurate to get information from a total group? In terms of practicalities, it will not always be possible to collect information from an entire group. For example, we can not send a questionnaire to every pregnant woman in Britain as many would have delivered before we found out who they were. It can also be extremely expensive to gather information from a total group, and it may not always be that much more accurate than a sample anyway. Polit and Hungler (1997) suggest that it is almost always possible to gain reasonably accurate results from a sample rather than an entire population. However, it is worth emphasizing that this will depend on the way the sample has been selected.

The aim of sampling is to select a sample in such a way that it has the minimum of bias, and represents the characteristics of those in the population as closely as possible. A biased sample would consist of people, events or things, who were very different from those in the total group. An example of a biased sample would be a study which used a group of pregnant midwives to 'stand for' pregnant women in general and ask how they intended feeding their baby. We would expect there to be a difference between this sample and the total population of pregnant women which would make decisions made on the results unreliable.

LoBiondo-Wood and Haber (1994) suggest that when sampling is properly carried out it allows the researcher to draw inferences and make generalizations about the population without examining each unit in the population. It is clear from this that the method of sampling deserves a great deal of attention. We should ensure that it has been planned in such a way as to recognize and minimize potential bias.

Inclusion exclusion criteria

Before we select our sample we need to define our population accurately. This is achieved by specifying *inclusion and exclusion criteria*. Our inclusion criteria are the characteristics we want those in our sample to possess. Examples of inclusion criteria would be women who have a normal vaginal delivery at term, or women in certain age groups with no complications of pregnancy. In other words, it is the characteristics they must possess to allow them to stand for the general group we want to say something about.

Exclusion criteria consist of those characteristics we do not want those in our sample to have because it may make them untypical and so bias the results. There may be other reasons for excluding some people from a study, such as the risk of harm for those with a certain condition or characteristic. Talbot (1995) defines exclusion criteria as characteristics which a participant may possess that could confound or contaminate the results of the study. In other words they will adversely affect the accuracy of the results.

The researcher must consider the inclusion and exclusion criteria at the planning stage. These should be clearly stated in any report for the reader to consider whether they could lead to some limitations in applying the results to other groups. A good example of inclusion and exclusion criteria is given by Alexander (1996) who lists the following for her randomized control study on the effect of breast shells on women with inverted or non-protractile nipples:

- At least one inverted or non-protractile nipple
- Nulliparous
- Intending to breastfeed
- Not intending to have the baby adopted
- Not already using shells or any kind of nipple exercises during the current pregnancy
- Between 25 and 35 weeks gestation
- Singleton pregnancy
- Had not had surgery involving the nipple or areola.

Sampling methods

At this point we must recognize that different research approaches will require different sampling methods, although some methods can be used in a variety of approaches. In any situation the researcher must try to draw the sample in such a way as to:

- Decrease bias
- Increase representativeness.

The aim of decreasing bias is to ensure that certain groups are not under or over represented in the sample (Couchman and Dawson, 1995). Where bias is avoided, or minimized, there is a greater chance that the results can be applied to situations other than the one in which the data was gathered.

What are the alternatives available? Box 12.1 outlines the main sampling methods available linked to the various broad research approaches.

Experimental sampling approaches

As we saw in Chapter 11, experiments have a particular function in research and that is to establish the presence of cause and effect relationships. In order to achieve this aim, sampling is carried out in very strict ways so that an accurate conclusion can be deduced from the findings. The method of sampling is drawn from a number of options grouped under the heading of random sampling methods. These particular options form what are called *probability sampling* methods. Using this approach, every unit in the population, whether it is people, things or events, should have an equal chance of being selected. If this criterion is achieved, it means that some of the sophisticated statistical tests can be used on the results. These allow the probable accuracy of statements made about the results to be calculated. Some of the alternative sampling methods in experimental design are:

- Cohort
- Simple random sample
- Stratified sample
- Proportional sampling.

RESEARCH APPROACH	SAMPLING METHOD
experimental	cohort simple random stratified sampling proportional random
quasi-experimental and ex post facto	cohort comparative groups systematic random
survey	cohort simple random stratified random proportional random systematic random opportunity/convenience/accidental quota purposive snowball/network/chain/nominated
qualitative	purposive convenience snowball/network/chain/nominated theoretical

Box 12.1: Sampling method by broad research appraoch

Cohort

For a probability sample it is possible to use a total group rather than a proportion of them, providing this is practical and feasible. Examples would include all midwives working in one particular unit; all women discharged over the months of June and July; the last fifty people who attended a particular antenatal clinic, etc. If all of these people were included they would form a cohort, which means a total group within certain parameters such as diagnosis, or time period. If each one was included they would have a 100 per cent chance of being selected which fits the criteria of having an equal chance of being included in the study.

In an experimental design the cohort could act as their own control group and receive both an experimental intervention, followed by the control intervention, or vice versa. An alternative would be the random allocation of half the group to the experimental group, and half to the control group.

It is worth emphasizing that there are limitations to the use of cohorts. A total group in one situation may have a different mix of characteristics to a cohort in another area. This would make generalizations difficult. Similarly, it is assumed in using cohorts, that one group will be much like another. That is, those who form a group in one time period will be similar to those in another time period. This may not be the case. Cohorts, then, have limitations in the extent to which they are similar to other cohorts and other periods of time.

Simple random sample

In many experimental situations it is not possible or desirable to take a total group as the sample, and a simple random sampling design is used instead. This is perhaps one of the most commonly misunderstood concepts in sampling. Many people assume that choosing a random sample is a haphazard, casual or indiscriminate way of selecting people for study. The word 'random' is assumed to imply that there is very little system applied to this process, which is far from the truth.

It is important to first of all differentiate between selecting a random sample and *random allocation*. In a random sample those eligible to be included in the study are identified from the larger population, and selected for inclusion in the research. This does not mean they have agreed to be included in the study, or that they will willingly take part. In the view of some researchers, findings can only be generalized if random sampling has taken place.

Random allocation, on the other hand, is frequently used in health service experimental research and is based on those who have agreed to take part in a study, and are willing to be allocated into either the experimental or control group. There is no guarantee that those who agree to take part in a random allocation research project are similar to the wider population. Random allocation is the system by which individuals are allocated to either the experimental or control group so that there is no bias as to who ends up in which group.

In order to achieve a random sample the researcher must have a complete list, or *sampling frame*, of all those who could be included in the sample. DePoy and Gitlin (1994) define a sampling frame as a listing of every element in a target population. Once the frame is constructed, each individual is consecutively given a number that can be used to identify them.

Individuals are then selected for inclusion in the study using a table of random numbers or list of computer generated random numbers. Table 12.1 illustrates a small portion of a table of random numbers. These can be found in many research text books, books on statistics, and it is also possible to buy books of random number tables. In all such tables there is no systematic sequence to the way in which the numbers are listed. That is, they do not go up or down in any particular pattern, or are listed in an alternating odd/even pattern.

12	57	42	14	01	84	35	21	75	33	61	68	32
85	83	35	22	13	38	47	90	15	65	74	40	09
10	39	55	86	16	03	91	75	62	34	11	59	17
22	08	60	13	26	99	71	40	91	69	35	04	65
49	74	26	39	09	16	87	56	20	54	88	93	82
36	06	33	47	98	49	07	19	51	27	43	71	54

Table 12.1: Example of a part of a table of random numbers

USING A TABLE OF RANDOM NUMBERS

How do we randomly allocate people in an experiment? Let us imagine the researcher has gained the agreement of 50 women and has decided to allocate 25 to an experimental group, and 25 to the control group. A sampling frame of the names of the 50 women is first constructed. The order of the names is not important. Everyone is given a number in sequence from 1 to 50. Then 25 numbers between 1 and 50 are extracted from the table of random numbers to form the experimental group.

The method of selecting the numbers can now be described. Without looking closely at the table of random numbers, the researcher puts a finger down on to the page and looks for the number closest to it. For the purpose of illustration let us say the number 83 has been identified. This is the second number in the second column in Table 12.1. As this is above 50, which is the number of people who have been allocated a number, it is ignored. Keeping the finger on the page, the researcher now moves their finger, right, left, up or down, or diagonally in any direction. As they move the finger each number between 1 and 50 is accepted, and any above 50 rejected. If a number has already been selected it is also rejected until 25 numbers have been drawn. So let us assume, having started at 83, we continue to move in a straight line to the right along the row. This would give us numbers 35, 22, 13, 38, and 47. Number 90 would be rejected, and 15 accepted. At any point the researcher may alter direction, or lift their finger and replace it at a different point. It really does not matter.

Once the 25 numbers have been drawn, those people who have been allocated each of those numbers will be identified from the sampling frame. These will form the people in the experimental group. Anyone with a number not included in the 25 drawn at random would be in the control group.

How would this work in the case of a randomized control trial where a sampling frame could not be constructed? For example, if people were to be selected for a prospectively study as they entered the system, say at booking or on admission in labour?

In this case the researcher would use sealed envelopes. The table of random numbers would be used in the same way as just described where if the researcher again wished to use two groups of 25 women, 25 numbers would be picked out, and designated the experimental group. A pack of envelopes would then be numbered from 1 to 50. In those envelopes, whose number corresponded with one of the 25 numbers drawn from the random table, a slip of paper saying 'experimental group' or stating the experimental intervention would be placed in the envelope. All the other envelopes would have a slip indicating 'control group' or the control intervention, or no intervention where an experimental variable was being compared to no intervention.

The envelopes would then be placed in number sequence from 1 to 50. As each person entered the study, the researcher would open the next envelope in sequence, and follow the instructions.

In the example of a table of random numbers it should be clear that the table used would only be applicable if the total number of people in the sampling frame was under a hundred. This is because as the numbers are in pairs, the maximum number would be 99. For larger studies, it is possible to use tables with three digit numbers which would be applicable for sampling frames extending up to 999.

Stratified sample

The basic principle of a simple random sample is that everyone has an equal chance of being selected for either the experimental or control group. There are cases, however, where that may result in an over representation of certain characteristics in one of the groups. So, for instance, the experimental group could have mainly primiparae women and the control group mainly multiparae women.

To avoid this the researcher can first stratify the sample into parity, and then sample within each parity appropriately. In the case of a prospective experimental design the researcher would use numbered envelopes for each parity. Once it is established whether the individual agreeing to take part in the study is primiparae or multiparae, the next envelope in the appropriate pile is opened. This way there should be an even spread of primiparae and multiparae women in both the experimental and control group.

An example of the use of this technique in a prospective randomized control trial is Drayton and Rees (1989). In their study, which looked at the routine use of enemas, one group received an enema, and the other group laboured without one. As the study tested the influence of the enema on the length of labour, it was important to have similar proportions of multiparae women in both groups, as their length of labour is shorter than that of primiparae women. The women were first stratified by parity before being allocated to either the enema or no enema group through the use of sealed envelopes.

Proportional sampling

A further refinement of the stratified sample is the proportional sample. Here, the selected number of participants in main sub groups is in proportion to their number in the larger population (Talbot, 1995). So with the example of parity, it could be felt important that the sample should reflect the proportion of primiparae to multiparae within each experimental and control group. If there was a proportion of 60 per cent multiparae women delivering in a particular unit to 40 per cent primiparae, then a proportional sample would also provide a sample with the same ratio between parities.

Quasi-experimental and ex post facto designs

Chapter 10 discussed alternatives to randomized control trials such as quasi-experimental and ex post facto designs. Quasi-experimental designs are used where it is not possible, usually for reasons such as ethical difficulties or practical constraints, to randomly allocate people to experimental and control groups. In these circumstances groups already formed are used. Examples would be women on two different wards, or couples attending two different locations for antenatal classes. One is used as the experimental group, and the other the control group. This is very similar to using two different cohorts in order to make a comparison.

The difficulty of this design is that it is not possible to rule out bias due to the blend of characteristics in each group. There may be important differences between the groups that may influence the outcome following an experimental intervention. Although this is a fundamental sampling weakness, in many cases this is the only method available. In these circumstances the researcher can attempt to illustrate their comparability by identifying and describing their demographic characteristics, such as age, parity, social class, etc.

As there is an unequal difference in the chance of people ending up in the experimental as opposed to the control group (everyone on one ward would have a 100 per cent chance and those on the comparison or control ward would have 0 per cent chance), this is known as a non probability sampling method. This is not as accurate a means of detecting true differences between groups as the probability alternatives described in the earlier sections, and for this reason it is less respected in comparison to the probability methods. It has the advantage, however, of being practical, and often the best that can be done under the circumstances.

Ex post facto studies, also discussed in Chapter 10, are very similar to the quasi-experimental approach in the sampling methods used. The term means 'after the fact' and relates to the formation of groups which have already taken place before the start of the study and differ in relation to the independent variable. The researcher does not introduce the variable, but looks for groups or individuals who can be allocated into groups on the basis of their own past decision to adopt a characteristic, such as smoking or deciding to breastfeed. Again this is a non probability method and we cannot generalize the findings to other situations with the same confidence as we can with probability sampling methods.

Survey methods

A far more frequently used approach to research in midwifery is the survey. Here some of the sampling methods already mentioned can be used and fall into both the probability and non-probability sampling methods.

Cohort

Surveys can first of all be based on a total group or cohort where all those in one particular group are sent a questionnaire, interviewed or observed. Examples would be all those attending antenatal classes in one venue, or all women giving birth to twins over a six month period. In survey methods, the strength of using a cohort is that it reduces the element of *sampling error*. If only some from a group are included in a sample, they may not accurately represent the characteristics of the full group. If everyone in the group is included this kind of error cannot exist.

The limitation of using cohorts in surveys is that sometimes total groups are just too large to include everyone. They also suffer from the assumption, identified under experiments, that one group is much like another, and that may not be the case. Factors such as seasonal variations or social class may make one group very different from another.

Simple random sampling

Surveys are very powerful where they are based on a simple random sample. Here everyone from the total population has an equal chance of being included in the survey. The method has been described above under experiments where a sampling frame containing everyone fitting the inclusion criteria is constructed, a table of random numbers is then used to pick out the appropriate number of individuals for inclusion in the survey.

The advantage of using this method is that it is possible to make generalizations concerning the wider population on the basis of a random sample. This is because it falls into the category of probability sampling methods. One disadvantage of this method, however, is the difficulty of constructing a suitable sampling frame where there are a large number of eligible individuals in the target population, or where no list of likely individuals exists.

Stratified sampling

The process of simple random sampling in surveys can be refined further be dividing those eligible to be included in the sample into appropriate strata and then sampling from within each of the groups created. Examples of this would include grouping women by parity, or in the case of midwives, grade, or length of service.

The advantage of a stratified sample is that it ensures that those from relevant subgroups are included in the study. The disadvantages include the difficulty of predicting which subgroups might make a difference to the outcome, and then the problem of dividing the sampling frame into those characteristics. For instance, if it was thought that women with high self esteem were more likely to breastfeed in relation to those with medium or low self esteem, it would be difficult to first divide the target group into strata by level of self confidence.

Proportional sampling

Proportional sampling in a survey would be an attempt to achieve subgroups within the sample which were similar in proportion to the broader population. The aim of this would be to ensure that an unrepresentative proportion in one group did not produce a biased result. An example would be a survey of midwives' views on a particular aspect of midwifery. To ensure that the influence of grade was kept constant the population would first be stratified according to grade, then the numbers selected from each group would mirror the proportion in each grade in the total population. Again, this example would use a sampling frame and table of random numbers, or computer generated random numbers.

The advantage of this approach is a greater chance of accuracy and reduction in bias. The problems are similar to stratified sampling, and that is the difficulty of having prior knowledge of the size of some of the subgroups.

Systematic sampling

In some surveys where individuals, or things, are being selected for inclusion from a very large population, systematic sampling is used in order to gain elements across the entire population. This is achieved by numbering all those who fit the inclusion criteria, then using a table of random numbers. The first number is selected randomly, and then individuals are selected following a predetermined frequency, such as every 5th, 10th or with very long lists every 20th, 50th or even 100th person or thing.

An example would be a questionnaire to a sample of women who had delivered in a particular unit over a three year period. In order to ensure that women from the whole of the three years were represented, all those discharged could be numbered, using a table of random numbers the first number could be drawn out, for example 48, and then every 10th number following that in the sampling frame would be chosen. So number 48 would be included, then 58, 68, 78 and so on. This would provide an even spread across the three years. Because the first number had been chosen randomly, it would conform to the criteria of a probability sample.

Cluster sampling

Where the elements in the sampling frame are geographically spread, or where the individual elements making up a population are unknown, a *multi-stage approach* called cluster sampling can be used (Burns and Grove, 1995).

Imagine a national survey of the opinions of GPs regarding how they perceived the role of the midwife in providing care for women in the community. A sampling frame of all GPs would be a tall order. Instead, the researchers may first produce a sampling frame of all health regions within Britain, and randomly select say a sample of ten regions. For each region they could then construct a sampling frame of districts. From this a total of three districts from each area may be chosen. The final sampling frame may be a list of all GP practices within the districts randomly chosen. From this a total 20 GP practices could be randomly chosen and all the GPs in those practices sent questionnaires.

It is clear from this example why it is called multi-stage sampling. At each stage a sampling frame is constructed, and a simple random sample selected. Each level consists of the construction of the next sampling frame until the size of the units is manageable.

The advantage of this system is that it can achieve an accessible sample from an almost impossible total population. The disadvantage is that the number of layers to the sampling process increases the degree of sampling error (Polit and Hungler, 1997). In other words, there will be a margin of error in the extent to which those left in the sample mirror the characteristics of those in the total population. Despite this drawback, its practical approach makes it a popular method in large scale studies that have a problem in drawing an accessible sample.

Convenience /opportunity /accidental sampling

These three terms are often used to describe the same approach to sampling where the researcher includes in the study those people to whom they have easy access, and who happen to be at the right place at the right time. Hicks (1996) also uses the term *incidental sample* to describe the same situation where the researcher selects the most easily accessible people from the population. This is the method used by market researchers where people are stopped in the street and asked to answer questions. It is this method which people frequently mistake for a random sample.

This, and the next two methods described below, fall into the category of *nonprobability sampling* methods, as everyone does not have the same chance of being included in the study. There is then no way of knowing whether those in these types of sample are representative or not. The ability to generalize from the findings is therefore restricted. Nevertheless, these approaches continue to be very popular because they are very practical in gaining quick and easy access to a sample, and provide an indication of possible responses to questions.

Examples of convenience samples might be women attending a particular antenatal clinic on a certain day, or midwives attending a study day who might be asked their opinions on some midwifery issue. The relevance of terms such as convenience or opportunity can be clearly seen from this description.

The advantage of this approach is that it is simple. It is also cheap, quick and does not require the construction of elaborate sampling frames. The disadvantage is that of sampling bias, in that those who happen to be around a particular location may not be typical of the wider population they are taken to represent (Talbot, 1995). An important point, however, is the extent to which there is variation in the population of the variable being studied. Polit and Hungler (1997) point out that where there is not much variation in a certain variable in the population, the risk of bias may be low, but where it is a very mixed or heterogeneous population the risk of bias is greater.

Quota sampling

This method is a refinement of convenience sampling as it attempts to produce a sample that is similar in certain key characteristics to the total population. The market researcher will use quota sampling by selecting so many people in certain age groups or occupation groups in order to argue that the sample is 'similar in structure' to the total population. In midwifery, there may be a similar attempt to include quotas such as so many women who are primiparae and multiparae, or in various age groups, or have experienced certain categories of labour.

In many respects quota sampling is similar in purpose to stratified sampling, but as Talbot (1995) points out, it differs from a stratified sample in that the participants are not randomly selected from each strata.

The advantage of quota sampling is that the researcher is in a stronger position to say that because the sample is similar to the total population, then the results may be reasonably representative. The disadvantages are similar to stratified sampling, in that there is an assumption that the subgroupings that may make a difference to the results are already known, and that the size of each of the groups is also know so that quotas can be calculated. It also depends on the information that allocates respondents to either one quota or another being easily ascertained from potential respondents.

Purposive sampling

This alternative which is also known as *judgmental sampling* involves the researcher handpicking those in the sample on the basis of the researcher's knowledge of characteristics they know the individual possesses. Although this seems like biasing the sample, its aim is to achieve the opposite and try to ensure that a range of opinions or experiences is included.

The advantages, then are that the sample is known to possess key characteristics which it is felt should be included in the survey. It is very practical, and efficient of time and money. The disadvantages include the lack of an objective assessment on the precision of the researcher's judgements on how far the respondents are typical (Burns and Grove, 1995). This makes generalizations from the results very difficult.

Snowball/network/chain/nominated sampling

This final alternative, which is discussed in more detail below under qualitative methods, consists of respondents nominating other individuals who may consent to take part in the study. It is used where it is difficult to establish who may qualify for the study because the inclusion criteria consists of elements that are either not easy to ascertain, such as an attitude, or are illicit or illegal, such as drug taking. As one person nominates another, the sample grows like a snowball rolling down a hill.

Surveys, then, can be based on a variety of sampling methods. Some of these will result in statistical precision where probability sampling methods have been used. In these cases reasonably large samples may be sought, and chosen from the wider population using random sampling approaches based on accurate sampling frames. The aim of this kind of survey is to be able to generalize the results to the wider population. Other approaches based on nonprobability sampling methods are less precise, but a lot easier to conduct. Although it is difficult to judge their accuracy, they can provide useful 'snapshots' of situations which can be used as the basis for action.

Qualitative approaches

As qualitative research differs in so many respects from quantitative research, it is no surprise to find that the approach to sampling is also different. Because the purpose is not to achieve a large representative sample from which generalizations can be made, sampling is not based on probability methods. The aim is rather to gather information from people who can provide inside information on specific kinds of experiences or who are part of a particular culture or subgroup. In terms of inclusion criteria the most important factor is that they have knowledge or experience of the topic or phenomenon under examination. Those who are part of a qualitative study do not 'stand for' the larger population, in the same way as quantitative research, they are included on the basis that they are a member of an appropriate group. For this reason, as Holloway and Wheeler (1996) note, the rules of qualitative sampling are less rigid that those of quantitative methods, where a strict sampling frame is established before the research starts. The main alternatives include the following:

- Purposive
- Convenience
- Snowball/network/chain/nominated sample
- Theoretical.

Purposive sampling

We are already familiar with purposive sampling where the researcher includes individuals, or events on the basis of the researcher's knowledge of their relevance for the purpose of the study. Streubert and Carpenter (1995) point out that in qualitative studies there is no need to randomly select individuals because manipulation and control are not the purpose of the exercise.

According to Morse and Field (1996), the two principles that guide qualitative sampling are appropriateness and adequacy. They define appropriateness as participants who can best inform the research according to the requirements of the study. Adequacy is defined as the ability to develop full and rich descriptive data on the phenomenon in the study from the sample units.

Convenience sample

Just as the purposive sample provides the researcher with relevant information, so the convenience sample within qualitative research is relevant as long as those at hand have necessary information or experience relevant to the purpose of the study. The convenience sample can be used in both phenomenological studies and ethnographic research where the researcher draws on the experiences and activities of those who just happen to be in the setting being observed, or under study. The appropriateness of this method again illustrates the flexibility in this approach to data collection.

Snowball/network/chain/nominated sampling

All of these terms can be applied to the situation where the researcher may identify some individuals who possess the necessary characteristics or experiences, and then asks these to suggest others who may be willing to participate in the study. This approach can also be used in survey research, as seen above. Holloway and Wheeler (1996) point out that this kind of sampling method is used where the researcher finds it difficult to identify useful informants, or where individuals cannot be easily contacted or where anonymity is desirable, such as those informally artificially inseminating themselves (Green et al., 1995). In many of these cases sampling frames just do not exist.

Burns and Grove (1995) point out that the advantage of this method is that friends tend to have characteristics in common and therefore it is a good way to collect a sample of people who share the characteristic under study. They go on to warn that biases are built into this sampling procedure as subjects are not independent of each other. This may not, however, be a problem.

Theoretical sampling

In qualitative research theoretical sampling is frequently used as a way of selecting the sample, and as a way of knowing when to stop data gathering. This is based on the principle that those in the sample can provide examples of the concepts or theoretical issues which are the concern of the research (Holloway and Wheeler, 1996). This helps to determine who will be included in the sample.

Data collection continues until no new insights are gained, and there is a repetition of information already gained. This is called theoretical saturation. At this point data collection is stopped.

Sampling in qualitative research is usually prospective and the researcher in ethnographic research will search out those in the setting it is believed will provide insights of use to the developing understanding of the topic.

Sample size

One of the most difficult tasks for the researcher is to establish at the planning stage how many people, things or events are going to be included in the sample. As the size of a sample is to a large extent influenced by the type of study, it is useful to consider the question of size under each of the headings already used in this chapter.

Experimental designs

As experimental designs are concerned with accuracy, there are some statistical guidelines the researcher can use in choosing a suitable sample size. The important factor is the size of the difference the researcher is looking for between the results of the experimental group and the control group before they are willing to say that an intervention has been successful. Unfortunately, for many conditions or situations, the difference between one group and another when measured on physiological outcomes may be quite small. This would mean that for differences to show up, the study would have to include quite a large number of people before that difference was clearly visible, and statistically relevant.

There is a statistical procedure called *power analysis* which can be used to estimate the total size of the sample needed, given an anticipated difference in the results between two groups (Polit and Hungler, 1991). Alexander (1996) attempted to follow this procedure in her randomized control trial of breast shells. However, as Alexander found, it can be difficult to recruit the large numbers that may be required to satisfy the statistical criteria for such studies.

For this reason, there are few studies in midwifery using experimental design, and some of those undertaken can be of modest sample sizes. It is often practical considerations such as time and resources that dictate the size of experimental groups. Closely examining the literature for the size of previous studies can be a great help to the researcher. It is also important to realize that it is not so much the total number of people to be admitted to a trail that is important, but the size of the sub-groups used in the analysis of the results. Where the sample is divided into differences such as parity, or age, the size of the groups can be quite small, even though the overall group might have been quite large.

One problem in experimental designs is the drop out rate from the study. This is referred to as *subject mortality* or attrition. Although the size of the sample can seem large to start, if the study is carried out over a long time period, or consists of several periods of testing and data collection, some people for one reason or another may be lost to the study. This can have consequences where there is a larger proportion dropping out of one of the groups as it can lead to an imbalance between the groups which may no longer be comparable.

The best the researcher can do is to try and make the size of the groups as large as is practical, and to ensure that the size is reasonably in line with any previous research.

Surveys

The optimum sample size in surveys is variable, as it relates to the size of the total population. In surveys where the aim is to be able to generalize quite accurately to the total population, the sample size may be in the hundreds. In other studies, where the total population itself is quite small, such as the number of male midwives, the sample may be quite small.

In choosing the sample size, the advice is to attempt to gain as large a sample as possible on the grounds that the larger the sample, the more representative it is likely to be (Polit and Hungler, 1997). However, there is also agreement that a large sample does not compensate for poor sampling methods (Talbot, 1995; Atkinson, 1996). The important point made by Polit and Hungler (1997) is that the ultimate criterion for assessing a sample is its representativeness. In other words, the researcher should be concerned with the quality of the sampling method and the extent to which it avoids bias, rather than simply including as large a number as possible.

As with experimental studies, it is often practical considerations which influence sample size. These include time, money and the availability of subjects (Talbot, 1995). This last point can be illustrated by a survey of interprofessional communication in a labour suite which used interviews as a method of data collection (Brownlee et al., 1996). In all, twenty midwives and fifteen doctors were randomly chosen to participate in the study. This was based on a total of sixty midwives and forty-five doctors. Although the total sample can be thought of as quite modest, in relation to the time consuming nature of the method, and the attempt to relate the findings to just one labour suite, the numbers are quite adequate.

The researcher should also consider the extent to which the variables included in the survey vary in the population. The more something varies, the larger the sample needed to gather a range of responses. The less something varies, the easier it is to capture the range of experience or opinion with a smaller sample.

Qualitative research

As we have seen throughout this and other chapters, qualitative research is so different from quantitative research that different considerations exist in almost all elements of the study, including sample size.

Holloway and Wheeler (1996) note that generally qualitative samples consist of fairly small numbers with anything from 4 to 50 participants. They emphasize that in the case of qualitative research it is not the size of the sample that determines the importance of the study. It is possible to find large studies such as Kirkham (1989) who observed 113 labours and interviewed 112 of these women later, having already interviewed 85 women during their pregnancy. It is more usual, however, to find much smaller numbers such as the 11 women included in the study by Bluff and Holloway (1994) which looked at women's perception of midwifery care during labour and childbirth.

Conducting research

In conducting a research project there are some important decisions that have to be made about the sample. One of the first stages is to be clear on who or what will comprise the sample. For this to be achieved, unambiguous inclusion and exclusion criteria must be developed.

The type of study to be conducted will influence both the size of the sample and the method of selection. In the case of an experimental approach a probability sampling method will be used with a reasonable sample size in each of the experimental and control groups. If relationships are sought but ethical or practical constraints prevent random allocation, then a quasi experimental or ex post facto approach may be used.

In survey designs the important decision is the extent to which there is a need to generalize further than the study group. This will influence the choice between probability and non-probability sampling methods. Where probability sampling methods are required, a sampling frame of all possible candidates for the study is required. This should be as complete as possible to avoid bias.

In surveys which do not require generalizations to be made to the larger population, and for qualitative studies, non-probability methods can be chosen. These are far more flexible and simple, and do not require a sampling frame of individuals.

In terms of sample size, the approach used will dictate whether a large sample of near a hundred or above will be required, or whether smaller numbers of ten or even less will be adequate.

When writing up a research report the researcher should clearly specify the details of the sample in the methods section. This should include the rationale behind the inclusion and exclusion criteria, the sampling approach, and the choice of sample size.

Critiquing research

In critiquing research one of the first areas to consider is the extent to which the inclusion and exclusion criteria may reduce or increase bias. What is the rationale given by the researcher for the choice of criteria? Using professional judgement, do those included seem more or less representative as a result of the criteria?

An important aspect highlighted by Burns and Grove (1995) is whether the researcher has attempted to generalize further than the sampling criteria would allow. For instance, have statements been made about all women in pregnancy or labour, when the sample consisted of only primiparae women, or excluded those of a certain age, social class, or other social elements?

Was the appropriate sampling method used in the study? The researcher should have provided a clear rationale for the choice of sampling method, and given clear details concerning the process of selecting the sample. This should be examined carefully to ensure that the correct procedures are evident. For example, if the researcher says a random sample was used, can we be sure they do not mean a convenience sample. There should be mention of a table of random numbers or other device if it was truly random.

In the case of probability sampling, is a sampling frame mentioned and does it seem complete? Has a non probability sampling method been used, yet the researcher has attempted to generalize to the wider population?

The influence of sample size should also be assessed. In an experimental design was there any problem with individuals dropping out of the study that may have affected the extent to which the groups are comparable.

If the researcher is clearly using a qualitative design, we should expect small numbers. We would still expect some detail on the sample characteristics so that we can judge whether they were in a position to provide information on the phenomena that forms the focus of the study.

The more detail the researcher provides on the sample the more able we are to judge the extent to which they have been rigorous in the way the study has been conducted.

KEY POINTS

- Research projects rarely collect data from a total population. Usually research is conducted on a sample taken as representative of the larger group of whom they form a part. This can consist of people, objects or events.

- A sample should be defined in terms of inclusion and exclusion criteria.

- Sampling methods vary according to whether the study takes an experimental, survey or qualitative approach. The approach to sampling can be further divided into probability and non-probability methods.

- Probability sampling methods allow generalizations to be made from the findings to the larger population. They include the simple random sample, systematic random sample, stratified random sample, the proportionate random sample and the cluster sample. In experimental designs, random allocation is more usual which relates to how individuals are allocated to the experimental and control groups.

- Non probability sampling methods include the opportunity or convenience sample, the quota sample, snowball technique, and the purposive sample. These are usually used in surveys and qualitative methods.

- Although non probability samples are weaker in design, as it is not possible to say whether the findings are generally applicable, they are easier to apply. In the case of qualitative research, it is not the purpose to generalize to a wider population, only to say that certain issues can be identified as relevant when considering a topic.

- Sample size is influenced by the nature of the study, the availability of subjects, and factors such as response rate. Experimental studies may be modest in size with 10 to 20 in each group, to quite large numbers such as 50 to a 100 or considerably more in each group. Surveys can be modest ranging from around 20 to several hundreds. Qualitative research can be anything from under a dozen to usually around 15 to 20. These numbers are only rough guidelines, and should not be interpreted as anything more.

CHAPTER THIRTEEN

The Challenge of the Future

The last chapter of a novel usually reveals all, and brings the plot to a close. It often has a happy or at least intriguing ending so that the reader puts the book down with a feeling of contentment, mixed perhaps with a little tinge of disappointment that the characters will no longer be a regular feature of their life. Non-fiction books are not like that. The aim of this chapter is to emphasize that what has gone before is only the beginning. This chapter challenges you to continue using the information in this book on an increasingly regular basis. This is not good-bye.

To consider the challenge of the future, the relationship between the midwife and research will be considered under two headings; the midwife as the producer of research, and the midwife as the user of research. These themes will be considered in relation to where midwifery seems to be going with research. It is intended that this final chapter should stimulate you to think about what you can do now, and in the future, to make best use of the information contained within this book.

Closing the credibility gap

'It ought to be a matter of genuine concern – to patients, health professions, politicians and taxpayers – that there is little, and often no scientific basis for most of the health care which is delivered under the name of the National Health Service. Instead of high quality research, the factors which dictate the content of much clinical practice are subjective or even subliminal. Most of what we do, we do because we do it; history, tradition, obscure and often personal notions of professionalism and unsubstantiated opinion continue to dominate a high proportion of decision making in health care. This is true of both clinical and managerial processes in health care, the latter no less culpable than the former, and applies to all the key professions in the field.' (Baker, 1996)

This is a serious challenge that relates to midwifery as much as other professional groups within the health service, including medicine. However, throughout this book there have been a large number of midwifery research projects cited. The continued appearance of further volumes in the *Research and the Midwife* series by Robinson and Thomson, and the research based practice series by Alexander, Levi and Roch, would also suggest that midwifery does regularly produce research. So where is the problem?

The problem is this: although the amount of midwifery research has increased since 1975 (Harris, 1992), it is still more of a trickle than a stream. A further problem is that despite the availability of some research, there appears to be a credibility gap between the amount that is produced and the amount that is put into practice. The challenge for the future, then, is to answer the following questions:

- Why is there apparently so little midwifery research produced on a regular basis?
- Why don't midwives make more use of the available midwifery research?
- How can we improve the situation?

Why is there so little midwifery research?

Just as in nursing, research in midwifery is a reasonably new phenomenon. The techniques and skills of research are still being refined. Articles are now concentrating on methodological issues such as which is the most successful method of collecting certain types of data. Fraser et al (1996), for instance, look at what women want from midwives and compare the use of questionnaires, in-depth semi-structured interviews, and diary recordings as methods of data collection. It is research like this which illustrates the developing maturity of a profession's research strategy.

One of the reasons for a lack of midwifery research must be the number of midwives with research skills. The Oxford National Perinatal Epidemiology Unit (NPEU) is one of the few research units which has consistently produced a number of influential midwifery researchers and research projects. However, there are now a large number of courses, particularly at Degree and Masters level, which attract midwives where research is featured on the syllabus. Strangely, there is an increasing trend to regard offering students an opportunity to carry out research as undesirable at undergraduate, and even post graduate level. The usual argument is that the numbers involved could lead to saturation, although there does not seem to be any evidence to support this. It is also argued that the quality of student research is so poor it is better to have no research than poor research. This argument is sometimes extended to suggest that it is unethical to submit those receiving health care to poor standard student projects. This, however, seems to say something about the standard of academic supervision rather than the ability of the novice researcher who needs experience in order to develop understanding.

At the moment there is a lack of midwives developing the practical skill of carrying out research. It is not the same to get students to critique literature or design a research protocol. Although these approaches to learning about research develop useful skills, isolated from the experience of undertaking research they merely serve to open up a new theory/practice gap in regard to research.

If more research is to be produced we must discover acceptable ways of providing an opportunity to develop practical data gathering and analysis skills. If this does not take place, then midwifery will continue to get 'caught-out' through the introduction of a change, such as waterbirths, without evaluating its effectiveness and safety aspects (Chapman, 1994). This means when suspicion is cast on the procedure no research evidence exists to justify its use. Under these circumstances it can take some time to collect retrospective information (Alderdice et al., 1995). In the meantime, the activity can still be vulnerable to suspicion and criticism.

Why don't people make use of research?

Where research is rigorously carried out, why isn't it reaching its target audience and influencing practice? The first problem is that sometimes the results of research are not published and therefore become difficult for others to access. Hicks (1993) found in her national survey based on returns from 397 midwives that although 65.5 per cent had conducted a piece of research, only a tiny six per cent had submitted their work for publication with four per cent of the total group having their findings published. This would seem to suggest that even where research is undertaken, it is not part of the research culture within midwifery to disseminate the findings in the form of a publication. Hicks (1993) suggests that the problem may not be the amount of research undertaken by midwives, but rather the small number of individuals who get their work published.

This question of the use of research by practitioners is raised by the Report of the Taskforce on the Strategy for Research in Nursing, Midwifery and Health Visiting (DoH, 1993) which considers the utilization of research findings to be 'a matter of urgency'.

Even where research has been disseminated, we cannot, as Rogers (1994) points out, assume that dissemination equals utilization. Hicks (1993) has pointed out that midwifery has a long and successful history, and individuals used to working on 'professional judgement' may not see the need to change what they see as successful, in order to make their practice more scientific.

The under-use of research in practice was demonstrated by Harris (1992) in her research on the impact of research findings on the treatment of perineal pain. Only 26 per cent of the 76 respondents in her study referred to research findings to support their clinical practice, and in only one case was that research appropriate to the population in question. She found that despite a wealth of published research on the subject, important findings were not applied to practice, while the majority of the reported ways of dealing with perineal pain were not research-based.

Rogers (1994) suggests there are many unknowns as to why staff do not use research findings, and asks:

- Is it the practitioners' fault for being unable or willing to read, believe and implement findings?
- Is it the researchers' fault for failing to identify relevant areas of research and failing to disseminate research findings to practitioners in a readable and understandable form?
- Is it the 'organization' or the 'system' which is failing to support, encourage and reward nurses and midwives for innovative research-based practice?

Rogers (1994) suggests that these questions are based on a simplistic notion that if research is disseminated it will be utilized, and do not recognize the complexity of the situation.

Further analysis of the problem is carried out by Brown (1995) who uses a communications model of *source - message - receiver* to examine the problem in nursing. He points out that problems exist with the quality of research produced by some researchers, and that the way the research is written with a liberal use of 'jargon' can form a communication barrier. The location of some research articles in journals infrequently read by the target group is highlighted in the model, along with the skills of the 'receivers' to translate the message. When it comes to implementing findings, Brown (1995) points to the tradition in the health service of inflexibility and the slow acceptance of new ideas. However, the pace of change appears to have increased in recent years, although not all of it appears to be research based.

One problem frequently overlooked is the source of some of the research publications, and whether they appear in specialized journals which the majority of midwives may not routinely read. A fear expressed by Hardy (1994) is that with the move of midwifery education to higher education, there is an emphasis on publications in only certain 'academic' journals which count towards the funding of academic departments. This can lead to the more mainstream journals being undervalued as a source for publishing research findings. Although this is true, it suggests that midwifery tutors are major publishers of research, and this is not wholly accurate. It also does not take into account the work done by MIDIRS (Midwives Information and Resources Service) midwifery digest, which includes summaries and reproduces articles from a wide sweep of mainstream and academic journals, making this work accessible to subscribers.

Hardy (1994) also points out that there is an anti-academic tradition within nursing and midwifery. Where individuals have not taken part in research they can be resistant to believing that research can be a useful tool to clinical practice, and are often cynical of the emphasis placed on research.

We should be careful, however, in believing that research necessarily requires change. It may reinforce current approaches, or it might merely indicate that there are variations in approaches possible which have similar outcomes. This is where the critical skills of the midwife are important, in being able to consider the research in terms of the three categories Hunt (1981) suggested are response options for the informed reader of research. She suggests that the results of research may indicate the reader:

- Should do something
- Could do something
- Should review current activities.

This is an important distinction if we are to guard against using research in an unthinking and dogmatic way. Research is merely a tool which has to be used in a critical way as the following comment from Mason (1992) demonstrates:

'It is important to recognize the limitations of research is not static, and findings may change over time: such findings should never be regarded as 'the truth', but rather as the most accurate statement available at a given time about a particular phenomenon. Research findings are best viewed with critical regard.'

How can we improve the situation?

Under this heading we need to consider developing a research culture which first establishes a clear picture of what is meant by the term research and how it can be used in practice. Too many people may well have a negative view of research, and feel it is all jargon or statistics. This kind of barrier can dissuade midwives from considering how research can be used.

It is important to have a realistic view of what research can do, and avoid believing that it ought to provide the answer to life the universe and everything. Sometimes it provides more questions than answers. This still allows us to clarify our thinking, and should not be seen as a failure of research. Perhaps we were asking the wrong question. Often research can only offer general principles which cannot be applied in every situation. We need to make research an accepted positive feature in midwifery and this will only happen if more midwives develop the skill to critique research and realistically apply relevant findings to practice.

How can we develop a dynamic research culture in midwifery? A useful model suggested by Fealy (1996) illustrates that research application consists of a number of progressive phases. The model (Box 13.1) is structured a little like Maslow's hierarchy of need, in that it starts at the bottom and moves up once the phase below has been achieved.

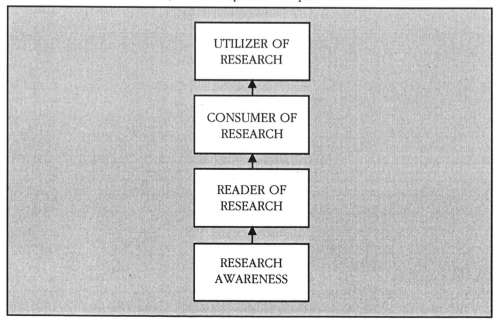

Box 13.1: Model of research application
(Source: based on Fealy, 1996)

The model relates to research knowledge and the individual, and starts with the development of research awareness. At this point the individual must believe that research has got something to offer practice. Unless this is recognized, the individual will continue to ignore research and see it as very low priority in making professional decision.

Once the individual recognizes the relevance of research to practice, the second stage is to become a reader of research. At this level the individual will take the time to read research articles, and may search for research to answer practical problems. At this level the individual tends to read research uncritically.

At the consumer of research stage, the individual becomes more discerning of the research read, and can differentiate between good research and poor research. It is at this stage that critiquing skills are learnt and applied.

The final stage of research utilization is perhaps the hardest of all. This is where the individual can take relevant research, and having assessed its worth, decide whether it should be implemented and where appropriate has achieved this. It has been noted in the literature that there are many barriers to research utilization. Even the term research utilization can produce difficulties, as Rogers (1994) found in her work. After much clarification, she defined it as a process directed toward the transfer of research-based knowledge into practice.

The importance of the model above is that it provides a progression of attitudes and skills which the individual can use to locate themselves in the hierarchy, and by taking appropriate action move up the levels until the final two have been achieved successfully.

The way ahead lies in more midwives developing research skills, particularly in critically analysing published work. This relates not only to single articles, but also the skill of producing a critical review of the literature. Both critiquing and reviewing the literature are high level skill activities which are developed with guidance and practice. In carrying out these activities, it is also important to use professional knowledge and judgements, and to be creative in the use of the available work. Do not expect the perfect research article to exist which provides the answer to the problem facing you.

An example of good practice in creatively utilizing the literature is provided by Walsh (1996a), who wanted to develop evidence-based practice guidelines for the labour care of low risk women. To achieve this goal Walsh used a number of sources including the Cochrane Database, the Alexander, Levi and Roch research based series on intrapartum care (1990), as well as a number of ethnographic studies including those of Kirkham (1989) and Hunt and Symonds (1995). The use of such a wide range of research literature requires a great deal of knowledge as should have become clear from reading the chapters in this book.

These activities must take place within a research culture, that is a supportive work environment that values the implementation of research findings, and where individuals are encouraged and supported to adopt new ideas and initiatives which are research based. Nelson (1995) has observed that implementing research findings cannot be left solely to individual initiative, and must be shared by all those working in the same environment.

Producing and using research

To develop a strategy to establish a research culture, we must return to the two alternative midwifery roles of producer, and user. Firstly, under the producer of research, it is important to emphasize that we should not expect every midwife to carry out research. Not everyone has the skills, or motivation, or availability of time to become involved in research. Yet someone needs to do it.

How do we develop a research producing culture? One useful development has been the number of midwives who have become involved in audit. This is only a short step away from research. The two activities are very close, and should be carried out with the same attention to rigour. The similarities are such that the midwife who has become proficient in audit has only to broaden the questions which drive the activity to become a researcher. As audit draws in the main on quantitative approaches, it would be useful to extend the repertoire of skills by undertaking a research course, either as a stand alone module, or as part of a Degree or Masters course.

More midwives must be encouraged to carry out good research. Hicks (1993) suggests that the reasons for this include the need to maintain professional autonomy and credibility as midwifery needs to develop a sound research base. She also believes it is important for midwives' own professional development and their credibility as a unique, discrete group. However, the most important reason, also supported by Hicks (1993), is to enhance the quality of care given by the midwife. There is a continuing need for midwifery to avoid complacency and to challenge routine procedures through research activity.

In terms of the midwife as the user of research, this book has already attempted to provide an understanding of the ways in which midwives can become critical readers of research. Although this is a useful asset for the individual, it becomes even more valuable where it contributes to a research culture. This means sharing the results of critiquing with others. Firstly, on a small informal basis with colleagues who may also be developing this skill, then, when more experience and confidence has developed, with a larger group of midwives. This can be as part of a small research appreciation group, or as a journal club (Aspery, 1993). Better still it can be a contribution to the work area, where critical reviews of the literature can be undertaken by small groups of midwives, as a basis for establishing standard for practice that can later be audited, or as a way of solving clinical problems or simply exploring new techniques and practices.

These are just simple suggestions; there are more creative alternatives which individuals should be able to develop. We do have to remember the barriers to change and remember that the best change may be in the form of gradual evolution rather than revolution. In other words, it is better to start in a modest way rather than have high aspirations dashed by a lack of overall support and commitment. It is better to start with a small group of enthusiasts and then work outwards.

If change is to develop, it must come from both initiatives from individuals and support from the organization (Hicks, 1995). This would suggest that the culture must include those higher up the hierarchy, including managers. Hicks (1994) warns that managers may see research activity, and support in the form of training, as a drain on the budget unless the benefits are clearly spelt out for them. Although she suggests that this persuasion can be an arduous task she makes this important statement:

> 'Nonetheless it is no longer acceptable to allow professional development in the area of research to be dictated by capricious provision or fortuitous osmosis; what is needed instead is some systematic training to enable the vast majority of individuals to learn and apply relevant research skills as a preliminary stage to making clinical practice more firmly grounded in scientifically derived findings.'

This call for action is a good note on which to end this section. The problems in midwifery research can be seen as a result of many factors. They will go on being a problem unless action is taken. The question is whose responsibility is it to bring about that change? Perhaps the answer is that at least some of it is your responsibility. Why not start now?

Conducting research

The starting point for research is to have a clear question that needs to be answered. The aim of this chapter has been to encourage midwives to think about their part in taking research forward, and one way is by undertaking a project. This does not have to be elaborate, time consuming or costly. Hicks (1993) has pointed out that one possible reason for the reluctance to get involved in research is the misunderstanding that to be of use, research has to be large scale, costly, and of earth-shattering significance. Small-scale projects, she points out, can have equally useful ramifications for clinical practice, policy and resources.

There are so many changes going on in midwifery at the moment that there is no shortage of developments which need to be evaluated. Walsh (1996b) reinforces the importance of this by saying that as new initiatives have been launched across Britain, the need to evaluate these changes has belatedly made it onto the agendas of the various stakeholders. In talking about the rush to introduce change in his own clinical area, he comments:

> 'In the enthusiasm to pilot the new, no baseline evaluation was made of the old. If this task had been undertaken, many of the dilemmas and difficulties in making a comprehensive evaluation of a multifaceted service would have become apparent at a much earlier stage.'

The warning here is that without research, midwifery could find itself involved in regression rather than progression. A great deal of damage can be done to long established services in the name of cost-effectiveness. There is a need for midwifery to be pro-active in demonstrating its worth in terms which managers understand, and which act as credible and persuasive evidence of its value and successes.

To carry out research successfully, it is important to have support from professional and managerial colleagues. You must possess a reasonable amount of research knowledge and have an experienced researcher who will provide guidance and where necessary supervision. It is always important that the project remains yours and does not become something your supervisor or advisor would really like to do themselves. In research, you also need a great deal of luck. It is probably fair to say there is never the perfect research project, and you must always expect the unexpected. It is a little like working with technology, if something can go wrong then it usually will. The compensation is that research is a truly exciting activity. Unlike the accusation that researcher's only find what they want to find, if you have designed your project rigorously and with the minimum of personal bias, there is no telling what you will find. And that's what makes it fun!

Once your study is complete it must be communicated. Firstly, to managers who may have sponsored it, and where possible to those who may have taken part, even if this takes the form of a one page summary, to let them know that their participation contributed to something tangible. If the study was completed rigorously, then whether the results were positive or negative a clear attempt should be made to disseminate it widely. This can be in the form of any or all of the following:

* A conference paper
* A conference poster
* A journal article.

As they are aimed at different groups, each has its own format, and serves a different function. A conference paper requires verbal and visual presentation skill, good voice projection, and a willingness to share your work with a group. Make it easy to understand. Use overheads or slides with key words or phrases and easy to assimilate tables, which are neither too small to see nor overcrowded with information. Overheads and slides allow you to talk around them instead of having to read from a carefully prepared script. Prompt cards are a good idea, but avoid a ten page script if you want to keep your audience awake.

Poster presentations are a good introduction to research presentations, as they expose you to the minimum of intimidation. These depend on visual impact, and gaining the reader's attention. Try and attend a conference first which has a wide variety of posters so that you can gain some good ideas. Don't forget to include your name and address on the poster so people can get in touch with you for more information. Brief summaries of the research which people can take away are a good idea, but again include your name and address. For both conference presentations and poster presentations, business cards, or even complement slips will be extremely useful, and will save you writing down your address for people in a hurry.

A journal article is one of the best ways to communicate your research to as wide an audience as possible. Mander (1995) suggests that this is crucial to research and should be considered as a stage in the research process itself. Journal articles differ depending on the journal to which you are submitting, as each has its target audience and journal style. Do not submit to more than one journal at a time. It is acceptable to re-work your article once published for another journal as long as it is not simply a re-hash. Focus on a slightly different theme. Don't try to condense a whole dissertation, or long assignment into a 1,500-2,000 word article. Just concentrate on two or three of the main themes. Make the article interesting by thinking of it from the reader's point of view.

If you are new to writing articles, seek the advice of someone who has already published. Co-authorship is also an alternative where you enlist the skills of someone with publishing experience. Always insist on your name going first, but you might have split any publishing fee 50/50.

The usual structure of all of these options of conference paper, poster, or article include the following:

- Introduction to the focus (what was the problem)?
- What does the literature say about it?
- What was the aim of your work (the terms of reference)?
- How did you go about it (methods and sample)?
- What did you find (results)?
- What does it all mean (discussion)?
- What do you recommend?

Whichever medium is chosen to communicate research findings, it is important to remember your audience, and the reason you are communicating. Do not perpetuate the myth that research is written in gobbledygook. Hardy (1994) emphasizes this by warning that the researcher may be tempted to appear 'scientific' by using research terms and concepts that require a great deal of prior knowledge on the part of the recipient. Where technical terms are used in your report, make sure that their meaning is clear to the novice. Remember, you were there once.

Critiquing research

In this chapter we should think not only of critiquing research but undertaking reviews of the literature (see Chapter 5) and implementing the findings where relevant. We also need to think about how we can disseminate the critiques and reviews of the literature to contribute to a research culture. This will not be an easy task, and we should be satisfied with a small group of individuals who can share our enthusiasm. We will not gain the support of everyone. A small successful journal club, or research interest group will be more satisfying and beneficial than a large group where only a small number bother to turn up, and you end up doing all the work.

Research folders, and research notice boards are a good way to disseminate information, providing they are regularly updated. Some invited speakers will also stimulate interest, but don't plan them for when most people are on holiday or there is something else going on. A guest speaker and three people can be embarrassing and hard work. I know, I have been that guest speaker.

KEY POINTS

- Midwifery research is now on the point of entering a new era of maturity. The challenge is to increase the amount of quality research produced, critically evaluated, and where appropriate implemented. The credibility gap between the amount of research produced and the amount put into practice should be reduced. For this to happen the main requirement is to develop a supportive midwifery research culture.

- There is a need for more midwives to develop the practical skills of undertaking research. There is no shortage of clinical problems which need examining, and new developments which need evaluation. More encouragement is needed for midwives to develop these skills, and support to undertake research.

- Once complete, midwifery research should be communicated through the medium of conference papers, conference posters and articles. These should be seen as a crucial part of the research process.

- One of the largest areas of deficit is the number of midwives who can critique research articles and produce critical reviews of the literature. When these activities are undertaken they should contribute to the wider research culture of the clinical area.

- The suggestions made in this chapter require someone to accept the challenge of the future. Let it be you.

References

Alexander, J. (1995). 'Randomized controlled trials'. *British Journal of Midwifery*, 3(12), pp. 656–59.

Alexander, J. (1996). 'The Southampton randomised controlled trial of breast shells and Hoffman's exercises for inverted and non-protractile nipples'. In: Robinson, S., Thomson, A. (Eds). *Midwives, Research and Childbirth. Volume 4.* London: Chapman and Hall.

Alison, J., Tyler, S. (1994). 'How to ensure research-based practice'. In: Chamberlain, G., Patel, N. (Eds). *The Future of Maternity Services.* London: RCOG Press.

Atkinson, F. (1996). 'Survey design and sampling'. In: Cormack, D. (Ed). *The Research Process in Nursing.* (3rd edn.) Oxford: Blackwell Scientific.

Baker, M. (1996). 'Challenging ignorance'. In: Baker, M., Kirk, S. (Eds). *Research and Development for the NHS.* Oxford: Radcliff Medical Press.

Ball, J. (1989). 'Postnatal care and adjustment to motherhood'. In: Robinson, S., Thomson, A. (Eds). *Midwives, Research and Childbirth. Volume 1.* London: Chapman and Hall.

Bannon, E. (1994). 'Artificial rupture of the membranes in spontaneous labour'. *Midwives Chronicle*, 107(1283), pp. 452–55.

Barker, P. (1996). 'Interview'. In: Cormack, D. (Ed). *The Research Process in Nursing.* (3rd edn.) Oxford: Blackwell Scientific.

Behi, R. (1995). 'The individual's right to informed consent'. *Nursing Research,* 3(1), pp. 14–23.

Behi, R., Nolan, M. (1995). 'Ethical issues in research'. *British Journal of Midwifery*, 4(12), pp. 712–16.

Behi, R., Nolan, M. (1995). 'Sources of knowledge in nursing'. *British Journal of Nursing*, 4(3), pp. 141–59.

Bergum, V. (1991). 'Being a phenomenological researcher'. In: Morse, J. (Ed). *Qualitative Nursing Research.* (Rev. edn.) Newbury Park: Sage.

Bick, D.E., MacArthur, C. (1995). 'The extent, severity and effect of health problems after childbirth'. *British Journal of Midwifery*, 3(1), pp. 27–31.

Bluff, R., Holloway, I. (1994). '"They know best": women's perception of midwifery care during labour and childbirth'. *Midwifery,* 10(3), pp. 157–64.

Bray, J., Rees, C. (1995). 'Getting down to research'. *Practice Nursing,* 6(8), pp. 18–19.

Brink, P., Wood, M. (1994). *Basic Steps in Planning Nursing Research.* (4th edn.) Boston: Jones and Bartlett.

Brownlee, M., McIntosh, C., Wallace, E., Johnstone, F., Murphy-Black, T. (1996). 'A survey of interprofessional communication in a labour suite'. *British Journal of Midwifery*, 4(9), pp. 492–95.

Bryar, R. (1995). *Theory For Midwifery Practice.* Houndmills: Macmillan.

Buckeldee, J. (1994). 'Interviewing carers in their own homes'. In: Buckeldee, J., McMahon, R. (Eds). *The Research Experience in Nursing.* London: Chapman and Hall.

Burnard, P., Morrison, P. (1994). *Nursing Research in Action.* (2nd edn.) Houndmills: Macmillan.

Burns, N., Grove, S. (1995). *Understanding Nursing Research.* Philadelphia: W.B. Saunders.

Campbell, D., Stanley, J. (1963). *Experimental and Quasi-experimental Design.* Chicago: Rand McNally.

Clegg, F. (1982). *Simple Statistics.* Cambridge: Cambridge University Press.

Cohen, L., Manion, L. (1994). *Research Methods in Education.* (4th edn.) London: Routledge.

Cormack, D., Benton, D. (1996). 'Asking the research question'. In: Cormack, D. (Ed). *The Research Process in Nursing.* (3rd edn.) Oxford: Blackwell Scientific.

Couchman, W., Dawson, J. (1995). *Nursing and Health-Care Research: A Practical Guide.* (2nd edn.) London: Scutari.

Davies, R. (1996). '"Practitioners in their own right": an ethnographic study of the perceptions of student midwives'. In: Robinson, S., Thomson, A. (Eds). *Midwives, Research and Childbirth. Volume 4.* London: Chapman and Hall.

Department of Health (1991). *Local Research Ethics Committees.* London: HMSO.

Department of Health (1993). *Changing Childbirth. The Report of the Expert Maternity Group.* London: HMSO.

DePoy, E., Gitlin, L. (1994). *Introduction To Research: Multiple Strategies for Health and Human Services.* St Louis: Mosby.

Dimond, B. (1994). *The Legal Aspects of Midwifery.* Cheshire: Books for Midwives Press.

Drayton, S., Rees, C. (1989). 'Is anyone out there still giving enemas?' In: Robinson, S., Thomson, A. (Eds). *Midwives, Research and Childbirth.* London: Chapman and Hall.

Eby, M. (1995). 'Ethical issues in nursing research: the wider picture'. *Nursing Research*, 3(1), pp. 5–13.

Feldman, H., Millor, G. (1994). 'The scientific approach to the research process'. In: LoBiondo-Wood, G., Haber, J. (Eds). *Nursing Research: Methods, Critical Appraisal, and Utilization.* (3rd edn.) St. Louis: Mosby.

Fielding, N. (1994). 'Varieties of research interviews'. *Nurse Researcher,* 1(3), pp. 4–13.

Firby, P. (1995). 'Critiquing the ethical aspects of a study'. *Nurse Researcher,* 3(1), pp. 35–42.

Floyd, L. (1995). 'Community midwives' views and experience of home birth'. *Midwifery*, 11(1), pp. 3–10.

Gans, J. (1982). 'The participant observer as a human being: observations on the personal aspects of fieldwork'. In: Burgess, R. (Ed). *Field Research: Sourcebook and Field Manual.* London: George, Allen and Unwin.

Garcia, J., Renfrew, M., Merchant, S. (1994). 'Postnatal home visiting by midwives'. *Midwifery,* 10(1), pp. 40–43.

Green, G., Kitzinger, J., Macaulay, L., Wight, D. (1995). 'Desperately seeking sperm: informal screening procedures'. *British Journal of Midwifery*, 3(12), pp. 641–46, 659.

Hardy, M., Mulhall, A. (1994). *Nursing Research: Theory and Practice.* London: Chapman and Hall.

Hauck, Y., Dimmock, J. (1994). 'Evaluation of an information booklet on breastfeeding duration: a clinical trial'. *Journal of Advanced Nursing,* 20(5), pp. 836–43.

Hicks, C. (1996). *Undertaking Midwifery Research: A Basic Guide to Design and Analysis.* New York: Churchill Livingstone.

Hockey, L. (1996). 'The nature and purpose of research'. In: Cormack, D. (Ed). *The Research Process in Nursing.* (3rd edn.) Oxford: Blackwell Scientific.

Holloway, I., Wheeler, S. (1996). *Qualitative Research For Nursing.* Oxford: Blackwell Science.

Holter, I., Schwartz-Barcott, D. (1993). 'Action research: What is it? How has it been used and how can it be used in nursing?' *Journal of Advanced Nursing,* 18, pp. 298–304.

Hughes, P., Rees, C. (1997). 'Artificial feeding: choosing to bottle feed'. *British Journal of Midwifery*, 5(3), pp. 137–42.

Hunt, S., Symonds, A. (1995). *The Social Meaning of Midwifery.* Houndmills: Macmillan.

Kenyon, S., Taylor, D. (1995). 'ORACLE study: midwives will play a crucial part'. *British Journal of Midwifery*, 3(2), pp. 75–78.

Kirkham, M. (1989). 'Midwives and information-giving during labour'. In: Robinson, S., Thomson, A. (Eds). *Midwives, Research and Childbirth. Volume 1.* London: Chapman and Hall.

Kirkham, M. (1995). 'The history of midwifery supervision'. In: Association of Radical Midwives (Eds). *Super-Vision: Recommendations of the Consensus Conference of Midwifery Supervision.* Cheshire. Books for Midwives Press.

Laryea, M. (1989). 'Midwives' and mothers' perceptions of motherhood'. In: Robinson, S., Thomson, A. (Eds). *Midwives, Research and Childbirth. Volume 1.* London: Chapman and Hall.

LoBiondo-Wood, G., Haber, J. (1994). *Nursing Research: Methods, Critical Appraisal, and Utilization.* (3rd edn.) St. Louis: Mosby.

Mander, R. (1995). 'Practising and preaching: confidentiality, anonymity and the researcher'. *British Journal of Midwifery*, 3(5), pp. 289–95.

Manley, K. (1991). 'Knowledge for nursing practice'. In: Perry, A., Jolley, M. (Eds). *Nursing: A Knowledge Base For Practice*. London: Edward Arnold.

Mason, C. (1992). 'Research in practice: rhetoric or reality?' *Nursing Standard*, 6(27), pp. 36–39.

McIntosh, J. (1988). 'A consumer view of birth preparation classes: attitudes of a sample of working class primiparae'. *Midwives Chronicle and Nursing Notes*, 101(1200), pp. 8–9.

McKie, L. (1996). *Researching Women's Health: Methods and Process*. Snow Hill: Quay Books.

Miles, J. (1994). 'Defining the research question'. In: Buckeldee, J., McMahon, R. (Eds). *The Research Experience In Nursing*. London: Chapman and Hall.

Morse, J., Field, P. (1996). *Nursing Research: The Application of Qualitative Approaches*. (2nd edn.) London: Chapman and Hall.

Moser, C., Kalton, G. (1971). *Survey Methods in Social Investigation*. (2nd edn.) London: Heinemann.

Mulhall, A. (1994). 'The experimental approach and randomized control trials'. In: Hardey, M., Mulhall, A. (Eds). *Nursing Research Theory and Practice*. London: Chapman and Hall.

Newell, R. (1994). 'The structured interview'. *Nurse Researcher*, 1(3), pp. 14–22.

Oakley, A. (1981). 'Interviewing women: a contradiction in terms'. In: Roberts, H. (Ed). *Doing Feminist Research*. London: Routledge and Kegan Paul.

Oakley, A. (1992). *Social Support and Motherhood*. Oxford: Blackwell.

Oakley, A. (1994). 'Giving support in pregnancy: the role of research midwives in a randomized controlled trial'. In: Robinson, S., Thomson, A. (Eds). *Midwives, Research and Childbirth. Volume 3*. London: Chapman and Hall.

Oppenheim, A. (1992). *Questionnaire Design, Interviewing and Attitude Measurement*. (2nd edn.) London: Pinter Publishers.

Paterson, J., Davis, J., Gregory, M., Holt, S., Pachulski, A., Stamford, D., Wothers, J., Jarrett, A. (1994). 'A study on the effects of low haemoglobin on postnatal women'. *Midwifery*, 10(2), pp. 77–86.

Phillips, R. (1996). 'Observation as a method of data collection in qualitative research'. *British Journal of Midwifery*, 4(1), pp. 22, 35–39.

Phillips, R., Davies, R. (1995). 'Using interviews in qualitative research'. *British Journal of Midwifery*, 3(12), pp. 647–52.

Polgar, S., Thomas, S. (1995). *Introduction To Research in The Health Sciences*. (3rd edn.) Melbourne: Churchill Livingstone.

Polit, D., Hungler, B. (1991). *Nursing Research: Principles and Methods*. (4th edn.) Philadelphia: J.B. Lippincott.

Polit, D., Hungler, B. (1997). *Essentials of Nursing Research: Methods, Appraisal, and Utilization*. (4th edn.) Philadelphia: J.B. Lippincott.

Porter, S. (1996). 'Qualitative research'. In: Cormack, D. (Ed.) *The Research Process in Nursing*. (3rd edn.) Oxford: Blackwell.

Rees, C. (1990). 'The questionnaire in research'. *Nursing Standard*, 4(42), pp. 34–35.

Rees, C. (1995a). 'A step-by-step guide to the research process'. *British Journal of Midwifery*, 2(10), pp. 479–82.

Rees, C. (1995b). 'Survey methods in midwifery'. *British Journal of Midwifery*, 3(12), pp. 652–55.

Rees, C. (1995c). 'Questionnaire design in midwifery'. *British Journal of Midwifery*, 3(10), pp. 549–52.

Rees, C. (1996). 'Quantitative and qualitative approaches to research'. *British Journal of Midwifery*, 4(7), pp. 374–77.

Robinson, J. (1996). 'It's only a questionnaire... ethics in social science research'. *British Journal of Midwifery*, 4(1), pp. 41–44.

Rogers, S. (1994). 'An exploratory study of research utilization by nurses in general medical and surgical wards'. *Journal of Advanced Nursing*, 20(5), pp. 904–11.

Rose, K. (1994). 'Unstructured and semi-structured interviewing'. *Nurse Researcher,* 1(3), pp. 23–32.

Rose, P., Parker, D. (1994). 'Nursing: an integration of art and science within the experience of the practitioner'. *Journal of Advanced Nursing,* 20(6), pp. 1004–10.

Royal College of Midwifery (1989). *Writing a Research Proposal and Applying for Funding.* London: Royal College of Midwives.

Royal College of Nursing (1977). *Ethics Related to Nursing Research.* London: Royal College of Nursing.

Royal College of Nursing (1993). *Ethics Related to Research in Nursing.* Harrow: Scutari Press.

Sapsford, R., Abbott, P. (1992). *Research Methods for Nurses and the Caring Professions.* Buckingham: Open University Press.

Sarantakos, S. (1994). *Social Research.* Houndsmill: Macmillan.

Siney, C., Kidd, M., Walkinshaw, S., Morrison, C., Manasse, P. (1995). 'Opiate dependency in pregnancy'. *British Journal of Midwifery,* 3(2), pp. 69–73.

Smith, L. (1996). 'Beliefs about the midwife's role in home and hospital deliveries'. *British Journal of Midwifery,* 4(3), pp. 135–40.

Spradley, J. (1980). *Participant Observation.* New York: Holt, Rinehart and Winston.

Streubert, H., Carpenter, D. (1995). *Qualitative Research in Nursing: Advancing the Humanistic Imperative.* Philadelphia: J.B. Lippincott.

Talbot, L. (1995). *Principles and Practice of Nursing Research.* St. Louis: Mosby.

Tierney, A. (1995). 'The role of research ethics committees'. *Nursing Research,* 3(1), pp. 43–52.

Too, S. (1996). 'Do birthplans empower women? A study of midwives' views'. *Nursing Standard,* 10(32), pp. 44–48.

Tucker, J. (1996). 'A comparison of routine antenatal care in Scotland in 1989 and 1994'. *British Journal of Midwifery,* 4(9), pp. 487–91.

UKCC (1992). *Code of Professional Practice.* London: HMSO.

UKCC (1994). *A Midwife's Code of Practice.* London: UKCC.

Walsh, D. (1996a). 'Evidence-based practice: whose evidence and on what basis?'. *British Journal of Midwifery,* 4(9), pp. 454–57.

Walsh, D. (1996b). 'Evaluating new maternity services: some pointers and pitfalls'. *British Journal of Midwifery,* 4(11), pp. 590–600.

Walsh, M., Ford, P. (1989). *Nursing Rituals: Research and Rational Action.* Oxford: Butterworth Heinemann.

Webb, C. (1991). 'Action research'. In: Cormack, D. (Ed). *The Research Process in Nursing.* (2nd edn.) Oxford: Blackwell Scientific.

Wraight, A. (1995). 'Writing a research proposal'. *British Journal of Midwifery,* 3(1), pp. 46–49.

Index